W0043204

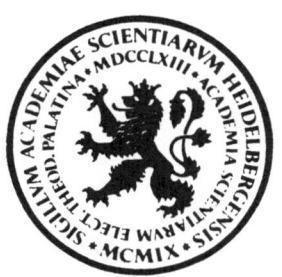

Sitzungsberichte der Heidelberger Akademie der Wissenschaften
Mathematisch-naturwissenschaftliche Klasse
Jahrgang 1989, 4. Abhandlung

E. K. F. Bautz   J. R. Kalden   M. Homma   E. M. Tan (Eds.)

Molecular and Cell Biology of Autoantibodies and Autoimmunity

Abstracts

First International Workshop
July 27 – 29, 1989, Heidelberg

Springer-Verlag Berlin Heidelberg GmbH

Prof. Dr. Ekkehard K. F. Bautz
Institut für Molekulare Genetik, Universität Heidelberg
Im Neuenheimer Feld 230, 6900 Heidelberg, FRG

Prof. Dr. Joachim R. Kalden
Medizinische Klinik III mit Poliklinik
Krankenhausstraße 12, 8520 Erlangen, FRG

Prof. Dr. Mitsuo Homma
School of Medicine, Keio University
35 Shinonomachi, Shinjuku-ku
Tokyo 160, Japan

Prof. Dr. Eng M. Tan
W. M. Keck Autoimmune Disease Center
SCRIPPS CLINIC and Research Foundation
10666 North Torry Pines Road
La Jolla, CA 92037, USA

ISBN 978-3-540-51436-7   ISBN 978-3-642-46681-6 (eBook)
DOI 10.1007/978-3-642-46681-6

Dieses Werk ist urheberrechtlich geschützt. Die dadurch begründeten Rechte, insbesondere die der Übersetzung, des Nachdrucks, des Vortrags, der Entnahme von Abbildungen und Tabellen, der Funksendung, der Mikroverfilmung oder der Vervielfältigung auf anderen Wegen und der Speicherung in Datenverarbeitungsanlagen, bleiben, auch bei nur auszugsweiser Verwertung, vorbehalten. Eine Vervielfältigung dieses Werkes oder von Teilen dieses Werkes ist auch im Einzelfall nur in den Grenzen der gesetzlichen Bestimmungen des Urheberrechtsgesetzes der Bundesrepublik Deutschland vom 9. September 1965 in der Fassung vom 24. Juni 1985 zulässig. Sie ist grundsätzlich vergütungspflichtig. Zuwiderhandlungen unterliegen den Strafbestimmungen des Urheberrechtsgesetzes.

© Springer-Verlag Berlin Heidelberg 1989
Softcover reprint of the hardcover 1st edition   1989

Die Wiedergabe von Gebrauchsnamen, Warenbezeichnungen usw. in diesem Werk berechtigt auch ohne besondere Kennzeichnung nicht zu der Annahme, daß solche Namen im Sinne der Warenzeichen- und Markenschutz-Gesetzgebung als frei zu betrachten wären und daher von jedermann benutzt werden dürften.
Satz: K + V Fotosatz GmbH, Beerfelden

2125/3140-543210

Preface

The 1st International Workshop in the Molecular and Cell Biology of Autoantibodies and Autoimmunity is convened at a time when recombinant DNA techniques have yielded the first set of data providing initial glimpses of epitopes recognized by autoantibodies.

It's aim is to bring together cell and molecular biologists with clinical scientists to discuss the broad spectrum of questions concerning the relationship between clinical symptoms and the specificity of autoantibodies.

The response to the call for abstracts was overwhelming: Nearly one hundred abstracts were received from many laboratories throughout the world. The topics covered by them are representative of the current research efforts going on to study cause and effect of autoimmune diseases. One of the aims of this workshop is to bring the rapid advances in the elucidation of the molecular structure of autoantigens to the attention of immunologists, cell biologists and clinical scientists and also to make molecular biologists become aware of the difficulties lying ahead in trying to understand the cellular and molecular basis of rheumatic diseases.

The organisers wish to thank NIH, BMFT and the Japanese Educational Foundation for financial support, the Heidelberg Academy for the Humanities and Sciences for hosting the workshop, Springer Verlag for their generous cooperation in including late abstracts in this volume, and, last not least, Ms. Simone KRAMBS for untiring secretarial help.

For the organizing committee: E. K. F. BAUTZ
                                                              E. M. TAN

Table of Contents

Clinical and Etiopathogenetic Significances of Autoantibodies to the Cellular Antigens in Systemic Connective Tissue Diseases

M. Akizuki

Department of Medicine, Keio University School of Medicine, Tokyo, Japan

Production of autoantibodies reactive with various cellular constituents is the immunological hallmark of systemic connective tissue diseases (CTD). The clinical significances and mechanisms involved in production of these autoantibodies were studied.

The autoantibodies were classified into two major groups: (1) those found in particular disease entity (anti-dsDNA, Scl-70, centromere/kinetocore, Jo-1) were designated as marker antibody and (2) those associated with certain clinical expressions observed in various CTD (anti-SSA/Ro, SSB/La, U1RNP) were defined as symptomspecific. The multisystem diseases which characterize CTD are explained by the combination of autoantibodies detected in an individual patient serum. Demonstration of specific autoantibodies has diagnostic and prognostic implications. Furthermore, the homogenous groups of patients were identified by specific antibodies: (1) antiphospholipid antibody syndrome: arterial and venous thrombotic episodes, recurrent spontaneous abortions (2) anti-aminoacyl-tRNA synthetase antibody syndrome: PM/DM with chronic interstitial lung disease and decreased lung volume (shrinking lung). (3) anti-SSB/La: patients with characteristic cutaneous symptoms.

Simultaneous occurrences of certain sets of autoantibodies gave us an insight to study the immunological mechanisms involved in autoantibody production. In addition to the previously known combinations (anti-Sm with anti-U1RNP, anti-SSB/La with antigroup (HMG) were produced in association with anti-histone antibodies. It appears that co-existing autoantibodies of CTD are directed to the exposed components of the same antigenic macromolecules.

Antibodies to the U1-RNP and SSB/La antigens appear to be produced by restricted B-cell clones and occurrences of cross reactive idiotypes of these autoantibodies were rare. These features are similar to those found in the specific antibodies elicited in experimental animals by prolonged immunization. Further studies concerning on the antigenic expressions in patients with CTD are indicated to explore the mechanisms of autoantibody production and pathogenesis of CTD.

Cloning of a cDNA-Fragment Coding for an Epitope Recognized by Anti-PM/Scl-Autoantibodies

M. Blüthner[1], E. Genth[2], F. A. Bautz[1]

[1]Institute of Molecular Genetics, University of Heidelberg, Im Neuenheimer Feld 230, D-6900 Heidelberg, FRG
[2]Rheumaklinik und Rheumaforschungsinstitut, D-5100 Aachen, FRG

Sera from patients suffering from Polymyositis-/Scleroderma-Overlap Syndrome (PM/Scl) recognize two major nucleolar proteins of 95 and 75 kd in Western blots.

Human HeLa cDNA libraries constructed in λgt11 were screened using affinity purified anti 95 kd antibodies. Initial screening of 2.5×10^5 recombinants yielded four putative cDNA clones coding for a 20 kd fragment of the 95 kd antigen, which on further analysis were shown to be identical.

Antibodies eluted from the fusionprotein recognized the 95 kd antigen in Western blot analysis and gave nucleolar staining in immunofluorescence.

EcoRI digestion of the recombinant DNA yielded a 551 bp fragment, which was subcloned into Bluescript vector. Subsequent doublestrand sequencing according to the dideoxy chain termination method showed one single PvuII restriction site at the position 240. To verify this sequence, the EcoRI/PvuII-fragments were subcloned into M13mp18 and M13mp19 and sequenced independently from both directions. A single open reading frame of the 551 bp fragment could be verified by subcloning this fragment into expression plasmids pUR 290, pUR 291 and pUR 292 in both orientations. The existence of the antigenic sites of the respective fusionproteins was probed by Western blotting with the PM/Scl-serum used originally for the screening procedure. Only the fusionprotein expressed in the correct orientation and reading frame gave a positive immunoreaction in Western blot analysis. All eight PM/Scl-sera tested, including a PM/Scl-reference serum reacted with this fusionprotein, suggesting, that we have cloned a major epitope of the 95 kd PM/Scl-autoantigen.

Fibrillarin from *Xenopus laevis*: cDNA Cloning and Expression During Development

M. Caizergues-Ferrer[1], B. Lapeyre[1], P. Mariotini[2], C. Mathieu[1], P. Ferrer[1], F. Amaldi[2], F. Amalric[1]

[1]C.R.B.G. du C.N.R.S., 118 route de Narbonne, 31062 Toulouse, France
[2]Università di Roma "Tor Vergata", Rome, Italy

Fibrillarin is a glycine-dimethylarginine (DMA)-rich protein associated with U3 RNA within a snRNP particle in the nucleolus of eukaryotic cells. We have isolated a 1.6 kb long cDNA clone from a *Xenopus laevis* library by screening with a DNA probe encoding a gly-DMA-rich domain in another nucleolar protein (nucleolin). The protein sequence deduced from the sequence of the isolated clone has been identified by comparison with that previously described for fibrillarin from rat and *Physarum polycephalum*, and is shown to encode the whole protein. As expected, the NH_2-end of the protein exhibits a 79 long gly-DMA-rich domain. Moreover, this protein also exhibits a domain that could correspond to an RNA binding domain, possessing an RNP consensus sequence. This result is in agrement with the fact that the protein is known to be associated with U3 RNA. The expression of fibrillarin has been followed throughout oogenesis and embryogenesis. Fibrillarin is accumulated during oogenesis and its expression is not under a translational control during early embryogenesis. Localization of fibrillarin during development has been studied by indirect immunofluorescence. Fibrillarin and nucleolin have been shown previously to be associated with the nucleolus in interphase, and during at telophase both are present in the prenucleolar bodies. We show here that, in addition to this localization, the two proteins exhibit two common structural features: the presence of both gly-DMA-rich and RNA binding domains.

Nuclear Receptors as Transcriptional Enhancers

P. Chambon

LGME/CNRS and U.184/INSERM, Fac. Médecine, Strasbourg, France

Steroid/thyroid hormone and retinoic acid receptors are ligand-inducible transcriptional enhancers which bind to specific cis-acting palindromic responsive

DNA elements. *In vivo* and *in vitro* structure/function studies using *in vitro* engineered mutants and chimeric receptors expressed in animal and yeast cells have revealed the existence of several functional domains responsible for ligand binding, nuclear localization, dimerization, DNA binding and activation of transcription. A model aimed at explaining how nuclear receptors may function will be discussed.

References

1. GREEN, S., CHAMBON, P. (1987): Nature **325**, 75
2. KUMAR, V. et al. (1987): Cell **51**, 941
3. GRONEMEYER, H. et al. (1987): EMBO J **6**, 3985
4. PETKOVICH, M. et al. (1987): Nature **330**, 444
5. WEBSTER, N. et al. (1988): Cell **52**, 169
6. WEBSTER. N. et al. (1988): Cell **54**, 199
7. BRAND. N. et al. (1988): Nature **332**, 850
8. TORA, L. et al. (1988): Nature **333**, 185
9. METZGER, D. et al. (1988): Nature **334**, 31
10. GREEN, S. et al. (1988): EMBO J. **7**, 3037
11. KUMAR, V., CHAMBON, P. (1988): Cell **55**, 145
12. GREEN, S., CHAMBON, P. (1988): Trends in Genetics **4**, 309
13. TORA, L. et al. (1988): EMBO J. **7**, 3771
14. PONGLIKITMONGKOL, M. et al. (1988): EMBO J. **7**, 3385
15. MADER, S. et al. (1989): Nature **338**, 271
16. MEYER, M. et al. (1989): Cell in press
17. BOCQUEL, M.T. et al. (1989): Nucl. Acids Res. in press

Multiple Components of SS-A/Ro Autoantigen: cDNA Cloning of the 52 kDa Protein

E. K. L. Chan[1], J. C. Hamel[1], C. L. Peebles[1], J. P. Buyon[2], and E. M. Tan[1]

[1] Scripps Clinic and Research Foundation, La Jolla, California, USA
[2] Hospital for Joint Diseases Orthopaedic Institute, New York, USA

SS-A/Ro proteins are common autoantibdy targets of patients with Sjogren's syndrome, systemic lupus, subacute cutaneous lupus, and neonatal lupus. Our aim is to characterize these components using immunoblotting and cDNA cloning. Human autoimmune SS-A/Ro sere frequently immunoblot a 60 kDa and a

52 kDa species in both MOLT-4 and HeLa cell extracts. In addition, rare SS-A/Ro sera also recognized a weaker antigenic protein of 49 kDa, which was distinct from the 47 kDa SS-B/La protein. From a λ Zap cDNA library derived from mRNA of human HepG2 cells, a clone Cl was identified by antibody screening using anti-52 kDa specific anti-SS-A/Ro sera. After several rounds of plaque purification and using a multispecific SS-A/SS-B autoimmune serum, affinity purified antibody to the Cl-encoded fusion protein recognized only the 52 kDa SS-A/Ro protein of MOLT-4 cells in immunoblotting. Bluescript plasmid pCl rescued from the λ Zap phage contained a cDNA insert of 1.5 kb and its restriction map was different from those of the known cDNA clones of a 60 kDa = SS-A/Ro protein and SS-B/La. Hybridization studies also showed that Cl cDNA insert was not related to the cDNA of 60 kDa SS-A/Ro and SS-B/La. Expression of pCl plasmid in *E. Coli* showed that it encoded for a 46 kDa truncated β-galactosidase fusion protein and, therefore, could represent about 80% of the 52 kDa SS-A/Ro protein. When partially purified Cl fusion protein was used as antigen substrate for immunoblotting, 7 anti-SS-A/Ro sera with anti-52 kDa specificity reacted with the 46 kDa fusion protein and its degradation products, 3 anti-SS-A/Ro sera with no anti-52 kDa specificity and other negative serum controls did not react. Southern blot analysis of human peripheral blood DNA restricted with EcoRI or HindIII enzymes suggested there are probably only 1 or 2 genes for the 52 kDA protein. Further analysis in the components of SS-A/Ro antigens may lead to an understanding of their cellular function and their relationship with the autoimmune response in these rheumatic diseases.

Autoantibodies to Nuclear Envelope Proteins: Characterization and Clinical Significance

J. C. Courvalin[1], M.-N. Guilly[2], F. Danon[3], Ch. André[4], J.-C. Brouet[3]
and K. Lassoued[3]

[1]CNRS, Gif-sur-Yvette, France and Rockefeller University, New York, NY, USA
[2]CEA, Fontenay-aux-Roses, France
[3]Hopital Saint-Louis, Paris, France
[4]Hopital Henri Mondor, Paris, France

Significant progress has been made in understanding both the function of specific nuclear envelope components and their biochemical composition. Macromolecular traffic into and out of the nucleus is now known to be regulated by an active transport system involving the nuclear pores and specific signal sequences. Pore specific proteins have been identified. The composition of the nuclear lamina, a proteineous network located between the inner nuclear membrane and chromatin, is now well understood. The three lamins of the nuclear lamina have been cloned, and sequence analysis has revealed that they are related to intermediate filaments. This relationship supports their roles as possible nucleoskeletal components. In view of their diagnostic interest, antinuclear autoantibodies (ANA) are the subject of intensive research. Autoantibodies directed against DNA, DNA binding proteins, ribonucleoproteins, enzymes and factors involved in nucleic acid metabolism have been characterized. Some of these antigens have been sequenced and their function(s) unambiguously demonstrated. In contrast, antibodies directed against the nuclear envelope have not been extensively examined, with the exception of those directed against lamins. We have been interested in this category of autoantibodies which represent a low percentage of total ANA (2 – 3%). 21 sera which recognize proteins of the nuclear envelope have been studied by immunofluorescence, immunoblotting and immunoprecipitation. They have allowed us to isolate two sets of antigens: the lamins and a 200 kilodalton protein.

1) The lamins:

11 sera were shown to contain antibodies to lamins [1, 2]. Sera from 8 patients contained autoantibodies reacting with lamin B, whereas sera from the other 3 patients reacted with lamins A and C. All patients (9 women and 2 men) had a chronic autoimmune disorder which does not fulfill the usual criteria for a diagnosis of systemic lupus erythematosus. Instead, the disorder was characterized by acute or chronic hepatitis, steroid-responsive blood cytopenia and cutaneous angiitis or probable brain vasculitis. Eight patients had at least two of these conditions. A peculiar feature of these antibodies is their high affinity and broad species specificity. Moreover, two anti-lamin B sera were found to be directed against epitopes which were also found in non lamin proteins, which may have intermediate filaments anchoring properties [3, 4].

2) A 200 kDa protein:

10 sera were shown to contain antibodies to a protein of 200 kDa [5]. This protein has now been identified as the major glycoprotein of the nuclear pore complex [6]. Strikingly, all of the patients suffered from primary biliary cirrhosis (PBC). As control serum displayed no reactivity, anti-200 kDa polypeptide antibodies can be considered as a new marker of this disease. To evaluate the incidence of such antibodies, 150 sera from patients with PBC were screened for the presence of nuclear envelope antibodies. 40 sera (27%) were shown to contain antibodies to the 200 kDa protein. We are currently searching for a peculiar clinical and histological feature which may characterize the subset of patients hav-

ing anti-P200 antibodies [7]. As these sera are both of high titer and affinity, they provide a powerful tool for investigating the function of this protein.

References

1. GUILLY, M-N. et al. (1987): Autoantibodies to nuclear lamin B in a patient with thrombopenia. Eur. J. Cell Biol. **43**, 266–272
2. LASSOUED, K. et al. (1988): Antinuclear auto-antibodies specific for lamins. Annals of Internal Medicine **108**, 829–833
3. CARTAUD, A. et al.: Presence of a protein immunologically related to lamin B in the postsynaptic membrane of Torpedo marmorata electrocyte (submitted)
4. LASSOUED, K. et al. (in preparation)
5. LASSOUED, K. et al. (1988): Autoantibodies to 200 KD polypeptide(s) of the nuclear envelope: a new serologic marker of primary biliary cirrhosis. Clin. Exp. Immunol. **74**, 283–288
6. COURVALIN, J-C. et al.: The 200 KD nuclear envelope polypeptide recognized by human autoantibodies in Primary Biliary Cirrhosis is the major glycoprotein of the pore complex (submitted)
7. LASSOUED, K. et al.: (in preparation)

Cloned Human snRNP Proteins B and B′ Differ Only in Their Carboxy-Terminal Part

A. van Dam, I. Winkel, J. Zijstra-Baalbergen, R. Smeenk and H. T. Cuypers

Central Laboratory of the Red Cross Blood Transfusion Service, Plesmanlaan 125, 1066 CX Amsterdam, The Netherlands

Autoantibodies against the snRNP proteins B and B′ are a common feature of the autoimmune disease systemic lupus erythematosus [1]. We screened a λgt11 cDNA expression library, made from polyA$^+$ RNA from HL-60 cells, with a monoclonal antibody specific for B and B′. This monoclonal antibody was obtained from a fusion between spleen cells of an MRL/lpr mouse and sp2/0 cells. Screening of 700000 clones resulted in three positive clones (clone 5, 9 and 16), which reacted also with a second monoclonal antibody specific for B and B′ and with a panel of human anti-B/B′ sera, obtained from patients with autoimmune diseases.

To characterize β-galactosidase fusion proteins, clone 5, 9 and 16 were introduced in a lysogenic host. All three clones produced fusion proteins with a molecular weight of approximately 140 kD. These fusion proteins showed positive reactions on Western blots with murine monoclonal and human polyclonal anti-B/B' antibodies. Human antibodies eluted from a blot containing fusion protein were shown to react strongly with B/B' on a HeLa nuclear blot. In addition, a weaker reaction of these antibodies with the A protein was observed. Clone 16 contained a cDNA insert of 914 nucleotides, containing an open reading frame encoding 252 amino acids. If the first ATG codon, which occurs in an nearby optimal context for translation initiation, is regarded as the initiation site for translation, a 240 amino acid protein is encoded.

From clone 5 a cDNA insert of 1049 nucleotides was isolated. This clone started 15 nucleotides more upstream than clone 16. Subsequently, 719 nucleotides were identical in both clones. At this position, clone 5 contained an insert of 146 nucleotides, introducing a termination codon in the coding region. Therefore, clone 5 encodes a 231 amino acid protein. A striking feature of the insert was the excellent homology with the consensus sequence for the 3'-intron acceptor junction for pre-mRNA splicing.

Clone 9 started at the 5' end at the same nucleotide as clone 5 and was identical to clone 5 apart from one non-silent mutation at position 359. An additional screening of a human cDNA placenta library, using a random-primed cDNA insert of clone 16, resulted in 24 positive clones, of which 8 clones also hybridized with a synthetic oligonucleotide complementary to the 5' end of clone 16. Restriction analysis of four of these clones showed that two clones comprised the 146 nucleotide insert, whereas the two other clones lacked it.

In vitro transcription and translation of cDNAs showed that clone 5 encoded a protein with a molecular weight of 29.5 kD on SDS-gels, whereas clone 16 encoded a 28.5 kD protein. Both proteins were immunoprecipitable with an anti-Sm serum and showed a difference of approximately 0.5 kD if compared with labelled HeLa snRNP proteins B' and B (29 and 28 kD).

To confirm that the two mRNAs corresponding with clone 5 and 16 were both present in human cells, an RNase mapping experiment was performed. Nucleotide fragments 665 – 899 from clone 5 and 650 – 738 from clone 16, obtained by restriction enzyme digestion, were used as probes. These fragments spanned the region containing the additional insert. The fragments from HeLa and HL-60 RNA which were protected were 233 and 73 nucleotides if the cDNA fragment from clone 5 was used as a probe, whereas the fragment from clone 16 protected a 87 nucleotide fragment. These fragments correspond with the fragments we should expect to be protected by the respective probes, if both the short and the long mRNA species were present in cytoplasmic mRNA.

From these results we conclude that B and B' differ only in their carboxy-terminal part, where B' contains one more repeat of a proline-rich motive. The proteins are encoded by two distinct mRNAs, which are most probably generated from one common pre-mRNA by alternative splicing. Both proteins are extremely proline-rich, especially at their carboxyterminal part. Homologies with the published sequences of the snRNP A and C proteins [2, 3], spanning six up to eight amino acids, were found. No homology with the D protein as published by ROKEACH et al. [4] was observed.

If compared with recently published cDNA sequences coding for a B/B' protein and for the related N-protein [5], our B clone was highly related to the B/B' clone as described. However, an additional guanidine residue in our clone lead to the introduction of a termination codon after amino acid 231, therefore shortening the protein by 56 amino acids at the C-terminal end. Furthermore, three extra amino acids were present in our clone at positions 172, 201 and 217, and amino acid substitutions were found at positions 5, 6, 173 and 218. Both B' and N contained 240 amino acids, with an homology of 92.5% at the amino acid level. Since the non-coding regions of the two cDNAs are completely different, these proteins must originate from different genes.

References

1. TAN, E.M. (1989): Antinuclear antibodies: Diagnostic markers for autoimmune diseases and probes for cell biology. Adv. Immunol. **44**, 93
2. SILLEKENS, P.T.G., HABETS, W.J., BEIJER, R.P., VAN VENROOIJ, W.J. (1986): cDNA cloning of the human U1 snRNA-associated A protein: extensive homology between U1 and U2 snRNP-specific proteins. EMBO J. **6**, 3841
3. SILLEKENS, P.T.G., BEIJER, R.P., HABETS, W.J., VAN VENROOIJ, W. (1988): Human U1 snRNP-specific C protein: Complete cDNA and protein sequence and identification of a multigene family in mammals. Nucleic Acids Res. **16**, 8307
4. ROKEACH, L.A., HASELBY, J.A., HOCH, S.O. (1988): Molecular cloning of a cDNA encoding the human Sm-D autoantigen. Proc. Natl. Acad. Sci. USA **85**, 4832
5. SCHMAUSS, C., MCALLISTER, G., OHOSONE, Y., HARDIN, J.A., LERNER, M.R. (1989): A comparison of snRNP-associated Sm-autoantigens: human N, rat N and human B/B'. Nucleic Acids Res. **17**, 1733

Antibodies to Ribonucleoprotein (RNP) from Autoimmune Sera Detected by Immunoblot on Tissue Extracts

E. Dayer, J.-M. Dayer, J.-P. Despont, and A. Cruchaud

Div. of Immunology and Allergy, Dept. of Medicine, University Hospital, 1211 Geneva 4, Switzerland

To establish the protein specificities associated with Sm, U1RNP, Ro and La antigenicity, 19 counterimmunoelectrophosis (CIE)-positive sera from patients with (4) mixed connective tissue disease (MCTD) and (15) systemic lupus erythematosus (SLE) were studied. Two SLE sera reacted with U1RNP and not with Sm. Immunotblots (IB) were performed on human spleen (HS) for the detection of Ro and La and on rabbit thymus (RT) extracts for Sm and U1RNP.

CIE		IB-RT (kD)					CIE	IB-HS (kD)		
RNP	Sm	68	48	46	45	28	Ro	57	45	30
6	0	6	2	1	5	4	1	1	0	0
0	13	0	9	11	12	12	10	11	9	4

Dissociation of Sm and RNP reactivity was best associated with the 68 kD protein. RNAse treatment of the extract removed the 68 and revealed the 44/42/38 kD proteins. Standard Ro antiserum reacted with both 57 and 45 kD proteins. Anti-La antibodies bound a triplet of 30/28/27 kD proteins on HS extracts treated by trypsin. In addition to the good correlation with CIE, IB on tissue extracts revealed the protein specificities associated with each antigenicity.

Analysis of the 60 kD Ro Protein – hY RNA Complex: An RNA Recognition Motif Within Ro Protein is Required for Binding to hY 1 RNA

S. L. Deutscher, M. R. Saitta, J. N. Kugler, and J. D. Keene

Department of Microbiology and Immunology, Duke University Medical Center, Durham, NC 27710, USA

Ro (SS-A) antigen is a common autoimmune specificity and exists in humans as an inabundant ribonucleoprotein complex (RNP) composed of a 60 kD protein and one of a series of small RNA polymerase III products, designated hY1-hY5 RNA. Detailed information on the structure and function of the Ro RNP is lacking. We have recently reported the isolation and characterization of cDNA clones encoding the 60 kD human Ro protein (DEUTSCHER et al. PNAS 85, 9479–9483). The Ro amino acid sequence contains in region of similarity to the

RNA-binding domain of the 70 K U1 snRNP protein. This region encompasses the octamer sequence which has been observed in a variety of proteins associated with RNA (DREYFUSS et al. 1988). In addition, Ro protein contains a potential "zincbinding finger" motif proposed to be involved in nucleic acid-or protein-protein interactions. The involvement of the putative RNA recognition motif (RRM) and "zinc finger" motif in binding hY RNA is being determined. Mutations in the RRM and "zinc finger" regions as well as mutations throughout Ro protein have been created. The recombinant proteins, overexpressed in bacteria or *in vitro* translated, have been used in reconstitution assays with hY 1 and hY 3 RNA transcripts in order to define the RNA-binding domain of the 60 kD Ro protein and to determine the stoichiometry of the complex. Gel shift assays using mutated Ro translation products and hY 1 RNA have shown that the putative zinc-finger is not required for binding to hY RNA or DNA. However, the octamer sequence within the RRM, is required for the interaction of 60 kD Ro with hY RNA. The sites on the hY RNAs required for interaction with the 60 kD Ro protein are being determined using various mutant hY RNA transcripts reconstituted with full-length Ro protein. Preliminary studies suggest that sequences at the 3′ end of the hY 1 RNA are not involved in binding Ro protein.

Monoclonal Autoantibodies Against Nuclear Proteins

S. Dyos, L. Alldridge, G. Dealtry, and M. O'Farrell

Department of Biology, University of Essex, Wivenhoe Park, Colchester, Essex CO4 3SQ, UK

We are investigating the role of nuclear proteins in the control of cell proliferation. In order to study the structure and function of individual proteins and also to identify interactions between different proteins we have initiated a programme to generate monoclonal antibodies to macromolecular components of the nucleus. We are using autoimmune strains of mice as a biological model system in which to generate monoclonal antinuclear antibodies. Splenocytes from NZ B/W F1 female mice (between 4 and 5 months of age) were fused with SP2/0 myelomas . Hybridomas secreting antibodies that recognise the nucleus of fixed permeabilised mouse 3T3 cells in an immunocytochemical assay were selected and cloned. Hybridoma supernatants were screened against growing and quiescent 3T3 cells in order to identify antibodies against growth-regulated proteins. All the positive clones were also screened by ELISA to identify, and in the current project, exclude, those clones secreting antibody against nucleic acid. We are currently characterising the cognate antigens of five monoclonal autoantibodies selected in this way. They are being studied in detail using immunocytochemistry, immunoblotting and immunoprecipitation in different cell types and different species. The results of these experiments will be presented. These studies indicate that this is a productive approach for the generation of monoclonal antibodies to physiologically interesting nuclear proteins. Knowledge of the range of nuclear proteins that can act as autoantigens will also give some insight into the nature of autoimmunity.

Alterations of the Macrophage System in Systemic Lupus Erythematosus (SLE) Developing NZB/W Mice

A. Emmendörffer, M. Müller, K. Hartung, and M.-L. Lohmann-Matthes

Dept. for Immunobiology, Fraunhofer-Institute Hannover, FRG

In SLE, a disease characterised by high titers of autoantibodies against several autoantigens (i.e. single and double stranded DNA) and by profound disturbance of the T- and B-cell-system circulating immune complexes result in a servere immunecomplex-glomerulonephritis. Since the role of macrophages in this disease is investigated only partially, our group examined the macrophage lineage in female SLE-developing NZB/W-F1 hybrid mice and agematched female BALB/c-mice as controls. We examined the animals at two different stages of disease, one group at an age of 6–8 weeks with no clinical symptoms (no proteinuria) and one with mice at a late stage of the disease with manifested glomerulonephritis. We isolated macrophages and macrophage precursors from different anatomical sites (liver, spleen and bone-marrow) and analysed their effector functions. The cytotoxic activity of the macrophages was tested against the TNF-sensitive target cell WEHI 164 and the TNF-resistant cell P815 in a ^{51}Chrom release assay. Microbicidal activity was investigated in a radioactivity release assay against ^{3}H-Thymidin prelabeled *Leishmania donovani* promastigotes. These protozoa are obligate intracellular parasites in macrophages. In addition, the macrophage precursors, non-adherent, non-phagocytic and NK-active cells were tested against the NK-target YAC 1. Further the secretion of TNF-α IL 1 and PGE$_2$ by organ-associated macrophages was tested.

Our rsults show an increased number of macrophages in liver and spleen and a up to 5 fold increase of macrophage precursors in the liver of the NZB/W-mice in comparison to the healthy BALB/c mice. The latter is already found in 6−8 weeks old NZB/W-mice. The cytotoxicity of the macrophages against the different target cells did not show any alterations between the two mouse strains. The macrophage precursors isolated from the liver of the NZB/W-mice were highly active against the NK-target YAC 1. This fact could be found neither in other organs nor in the comparable compartments of the BALB/c mice. The bone-marrow of the SLE-prone mice did not show any alterations in comparison with the healthy control. Regarding secretory functions of the macrophages preliminary results show a decreased PGE_2-production of splenic macrophages of the SLE-prone mice. TNF-a and IL-1 secretion revealed no significant differences between both mouse strains. Our results implicate a liver-associated proliferation and enlargement of the macrophage system in SLE-developing NZB/W-mice. This work was supported by SFB 244, project A5.

Cytoskeletal Proteins: Major Antigens in Autoimmune Diseases

W. W. Franke[1], L. Jahn[1,2], U. A. Simanowski[2], and G. Bruder[3]

[1] Institute of Cell and Tumor Biologie, German Cancer Research Center, 6900 Heidelberg, FRG
[2] Dept. of Internal Medicine, University of Heidelberg, 6900 Heidelberg, FRG
[3] Progen Biotechnics, 6900 Heidelberg, FRG

A group of "insoluble" intracellular structures characterized by their remarkable resistance to extractions in solutions of a wide range of ionic strength and pH values as well as in non-denaturing detergents, commonly referred to as the "cytoskeleton", are formed by different families of proteins, including cytoplasmic as well as nuclear representatives. Although these proteins, or at least most of their structure, are not exposed to the immune system, as long as the cells are intact, autoantibodies to such cytoskeletal proteins are frequently found in sera of patients with certain diseases; on the other hand antibodies to specific cytoskeletal proteins are also found, sometimes in considerable titers, in sera from apparently healthy persons and animals. The reported levels of autoantibodies to diverse types of cytoskeletal proteins (intermediate filament proteins, including nuclear lamins, 1−5; actins; tubulins; membrane-associated plaque proteins such as the desmoglein of desmosomes, 6−8, the M_r 220000 bullous pemphigoid antigen of "hemidesmosomes", 9, but also xanthine oxidase, 10) will be discussed in relation to the patterns of diseases in which their concentrations are frequently elevated. In addition, emphasis will be placed on the discussion of autoantibodies to certain cytoskeletal proteins that seem to be causally related to the origin and progression of a disease such as certain pemphigus antigens [11] and of the enigma of apparently "constitutive" autoantibodies to certain proteins in normal mammals, using xanthine oxidase antibodies as a particularly well studied example [12]. The experimental observations of autoantibodies to cytoskeletal proteins in both diseased and normal persons are also discussed in relation to the different hypotheses proposed for their possible biological and pathogenic functions (e.g., 13, 14).

References

1. FRANKE, W. W. (1987): Nuclear lamins and cytoplasmic intermediate filament proteins: a growing multigene family. Cell **48**, 3−4
2. KURKI, P., VIRTANEN, I., LEHTO, V.-P., ALFTHAN, O., SALASPURO, M. (1984): Antibodies to cytokeratin filaments in patients with alcoholic liver disease. Alcohol. Clin. Exp. Res. **8**, 212−215
3. KURKI, P., VIRTANEN, I. (1985): The detection of smooth muscle antibodies reacting with intermediate filaments of desmin type. Journal of Immunological Methods **76**, 329−335
4. GALBRAITH, G. M. P, EMERSON, D., FUDENBERG, H. H., GIBBS, C. J., GAJDUSEK, D. C. (1986): Antibodies to neurofilament protein in retinitis pigmentosa. J. Clin. Invest. **78**, 865−869
5. IWATSUKI, K., VIAC, J., REANO, A., MORERA, A., STAQUET, M.-J., THIVOLET, J., MONIER, J.-C. (1986): Comparative studies on naturally occurring antikeratin antibodies in human sera. J. Invest. Dermatol. **87**, 179−184
6. FRANKE, W. W., COWIN, P., SCHMELZ, M., KAPPRELL, H.-P. (1987): The desmosomal plaque and the cytoskeleton. In: Junctional Complexes of Epithelial Cells. Ciba Foundation Symposium 125. Wiley & Sons, Chichester, pp. 26−44
7. KOULU, L., KUSUMI, A., STEINBERG, M. S., KLAUS-KOVTUN, V., STANLEY, J. R. (1984) Human autoantibodies against a desmosomal core protein in pemphigus foliaceus. J. Exp. Med. **160**, 1509−1518
8. MATIS, W. L., ANHALT, G. J., DIAZ, L. A., RIVITTI, E. A., MARTINS, C. R., BERGER, R. S. (1987): Calcium enhances the sensitivity of immunofluorescence for pemphigus antibodies. J. Invest. Dermatol. **89**, 302−304
9. STANLEY, J. R., TANAKA, T., MUELLER, S., KLAUS-KOVTUN, V., ROOP, D. (1988): Isolation of complementary DNA for bullous pemphigoid antigen by use of patients' autoantibodies. J. Clin. Invest. **82**, 1864−1870
10. JARASCH, E.-D., GRUND, C., BRUDER, G., HEID, H. W., KEENAN, T. W., FRANKE, W. W. (1981): Localization of xanthine oxidase in mammary gland epithelium and capillary endothelium. Cell **25**, 67−82
11. ANHALT, G. J., LABIB, R. S., VOORHEES, J. J., BEALS, T. F., DIAZ, L. A. (1982): Induction of pemphigus in neonatal mice by passive transfer of IgG from patients with the disease. N. Engl. J. Med. **106**, 1189−1196

12. BRUDER, G., JARASCH, E.-D., HEID, H. W. (1984): High concentrations of antibodies to Xanthine oxidase in human and animal sera. J. Clin. Invest. **74**, 783–794

13. COHEN, I. R., COOKE, A. (1986): Natural autoantibodies might prevent autoimmunue disease. Immunol. Today **7**, 363–364

14. HANSSON, G. K., LAGERSTEDT, E., BENGTSSON, A., HEIDEMAN, M. (1987): IgB binding to cytoskeletal intermediate filaments activates the complement cascade. Exp. Cell Res. **170**, 338–350

Leucine Periodicity of U2 snRNP Autoantigen A' Implicated in U2 snRNP Protein: Protein Interactions

L. D. Fresco and J. D. Keene

Department of Microbiology and Immunology, Duke University Medical Center Durham, North Carolina, USA

A' is unique protein component of the U2 class of U snRNPs that mediate splicing in metazoan nuclei. Moreover, it is an autoantigen recognized by a rare subset of autoimmune sera directed against unique epitopes of the U2 snRNP. Anti-(U2) RNP autoantibodies, reactive with U2 RNP-specific proteins A' and B'', occur in patients with rheumatic overlap syndromes that include myositis as a common feature.

To gain further insight into the structure of the U2 snRNP and to facilitate analysis of the structural basis of its function, the cDNA and gene encoding human A' were cloned and analyzed using a (U1/U2) RNP human autoantiserum as the initial probe. Analysis of A' mRNA and a corresponding genomic clone demonstrated that the A' gene, spanning almost 20 Kb, encompasses nine exons. A putative regulatory region that is reminiscent of many constitutively expressed "housekeeping" genes resides upstream of the transcription start site. The primary structures of various cDNA clones recovered from libraries of different tissues suggest that two different isoforms arise by alternative splicing of the primary A' mRNA. Sequence analysis of a full-length cDNA disclosed an ORF that encodes a 225 amino acid protein of 28,419 Da.

To explore the role of snRNP proteins in splicing and to study snRNP assembly, we have initially reconstituted the U2 snRNP complex using wild type and mutant forms of A'. Upon incubation in a HeLa cell nuclear extract, *in vitro* synthesized A' was able to assemble into a U2 snRNP, either by exchange or by de *novo* assembly, as defined by particle density and coimmunoprecipitation. To delineate the limits of the A' polypeptide required for this reconstitution, association of N-terminal and C-terminal deletion mutants of A' was examined. The required region encompassed a portion of the molecule that displays significant internal homology. This segment comprises at least five approximately 24 amino acid tandem repeats that exhibit a periodicity of leucine and asparagine residues. This repeated motif, distinct from the "leucine zipper", is conserved in a wide array of proteins with diverse biological roles whose common feature is a role in protein: protein interactions: mammalian RNase/angiogenin inhibitors; the subunits of the human platelet integral plasma membrane heterodimer, FGIb; the proteoglycan core proteins of human placenta fibroblasts, PG40, and bovine bone, PG-II; Drosophila *Toll* gene product that specifies dorsal-ventral polarity of the early embryo; Drosophila chaoptin, a cell surface glycoprotein; and yeast adenylate cyclase. Occurrence of this motif in species from yeast to human implies that this element defines a widely utilized structural motif that presumably functions in protein: protein interactions. Unique regions of A' feature sequence similarity to the 50S ribosomal protein L1 of *E. coli* and a highly acidic hydrophilic C-terminal tail, which appear to be non-essential for association with the U2 snRNP. Autoantigenic epitopes reside in both N-terminal and C-terminal regions of the molecule. A' provides the first example of a nuclear protein that possesses a leucine-rich amphipathic repeat motif, and the requirement of this region for association with the U2 snRNP is compatible with a role in protein: protein interactions. Currently, we are testing the proposal that the repeated motify mediates specific protein: protein interactions of the U2 snRNP wihtin the spliceosome.

Epitope Mapping of the Recombinant Human U1snRNP 68 k Protein

H. Fujii[1], K. Yamamoto[1], H. Kohsaka[1], Y. Tanaka[1], H. Miura[1], Y. Misaki[1], K. Nishioka[2], and T. Miyamoto[1]

[1]Department of Medicine and Physical Therapy, Faculty of Medicine, University of Tokyo, Japan
[2]Institute of Rheumatology, Tokyo Women's Medical College, Tokyo, Japan

U1snRNP 68 k protein is a major target molecule of anti-RNP antibodies found in mixed connective tissue disease and other autoimmune diseases. In order to investigate the mechanisms of autoantibody production and pathogenesis, we have screened two different human cDNA libraries (fibroblast and fore skin) using a cDNA clone FL70K (kindly supplied by Drs. LÜHRMANN and PHILIPSON).

The longest cDNA clone (FR68) was about 1.7 kb in length which corresponded to the length of the band obtained in the Northern blot analysis using HeLa cell RNA. The cDNA was subcloned into a plasmid expression vector pEX-3 and positive clones were screened using anti-RNP positive patients' sera. The recombinant plasmid (FR68EX) expressed a fusion protein with cro-β-galactosidase whose molecular weight was estimated to be about 170 kDa. To determine the epitope(s), many in-frame deletion mutants were produced using restriction sites within cDNA or by digestion with exonuclease III. The resultant fusion proteins were partially purified and applied for the enzyme linked immunosorbent assay' (ELISA). Three-fourth of conventionally determined anti-RNP positive sera were shown to be positive.

The cDNA clone FR68EX contains an insert of 1.7 kb which is identical with the 3' terminal half of FL70K (THEISSEN et al. EMBO J. 1986) and contains a probable initiation codon located at 1212 of FL70K, which is consistent with Spritz' argument that the initiation codon of the functional mRNA of the 68 k protein is not located at nucleotide position 681 but at 1212 (NAR. 1987). Deletion mutants of FR68EX express fusion proteins with different molecular weights ranging from 116 kDa (cro-β-galactosidase) to 170 kDa (FR68EX), which were stained with several anti-RNP positive sera. Deletion mutants which contain more than 600 bp from the initiation codon show comparably positive staining to that obtained with FR68EX, but a deletion mutant which contains only 5'-terminal 150 bp shows negative staining. Thus, we tentatively concluded that at least one of the major epitopes resides between nucleotide positions 1363 and 1803. This region contains a nucleotide sequence encoding amino acids homologous to that of murine leukemia virus group-specific antigen $p^{30\,gag}$ (KEENE et al. Cell. 1987).

Molecular Characterization of the PM/SCL Antigen

C. Gelpi, A. Algueró, Ma. A. Martinez, S. Vidal, C. Juárez,
and J. L. Rodríguez-Sánchez

Hospital de la Santa Creu i Sant Pau, Hospital Universitari de la Facultat de Medicina de la Universitat Autónoma de Barcelona, San Antonio Ma. Claret, 167, 08025 Barcelona, Spain

In the 117 sera study of patients with progressive systemic scleroderma (72) polimyositis (12) and sclero-polimyositis (23), 12 precipitated a macromolecular complex of 13 polypeptides, whose aproximate molecular weights were: 110, 90,

80, 64, 47, 46, 40, 37, 33, 30, 27, 26, 22, 20, and 18 kDa. This complex was identified with the PM/Scl antigen by its electrophoretic pattern equal to that given by a control reference serum kindly provided by Eng Tan. Of these proteins, those of 64 and 40 kDa were in a phosphorylated form.

When studied by IIF on Hep-2 and HeLa cells cultivated on slides, each serum showed a fluorescent pattern mainly nucleolar and weakly granular in the nucleoplasm. The cells' cytoplasm also showed a weak fluorescence preferentially with a perinuclear localization.

These sera were studied by following the immunoblotting technique on HeLa and FLC cell extracts and on isolated nucleolus and nucleolar chromatine extracts of these same cells. All the sera, including the reference serum, recognized the 110 kDa molecular weight polypeptide. This was the same protein that manifested the nucleolar and nucleoplasmic fluorescent pattern, since the antibodies affinity purified by elution from the nitrocellulose paper (IB), afforded the same fluorescence pattern as the sera. When the antibodies were studied by IB on nucleoli extracts and on total HeLa and FLC cell extracts, they recognized the same reactive 110 kDa peptide. Finally, we demonstrated that the 110 kDa polypeptide, carrier of the epitopes recognized by the anti-PM/Scl antibodies is the same one that, with this same molecular weight, forms part of the macromolecular complex immunoprecipitated by these antibodies.

In the study of the snRNAs precipitated by these sera, only small quantities of rRNA were detected in each case.

The enzymatic digestions with DNase, RNase and trypsin of the cells employed for the IIF, demonstrated that this antigen was resistant to digestion with DNase and RNase and sensitive to treatment with trypsin. On the other hand, after treating the cultivated cells with Actinomycin D, with concentrations capable of inhibiting the action of the RNA pol. I, the antigen appeared localized in the nucleoplasm of the cell.

Upon treating the extracts employed for the IB studies of this antigen with DNase, RNase, and trypsin, it was observed that the reaction of the sera with the 110 kDa protein is sensitive to the action of DNase and of trypsin. On the other hand, after treating with DNase the complex precipitated by the anti-PM/Scl antibodies, the 110 kDa protein did not appear in the SDS-PAGE gel employed for the electrophoretic analysis of these proteins.

Finally, the results obtained by immunoprecipitation of total cell extracts and isolated nucleoli extracts allow the hypothesis of the existance of two macromolecular forms of the antigen to be postulated; one constituted by the aforementioned 13 polypeptides, and the other, enriched in the 110 kDa protein with a preferential nucleolar localization.

The results of the redistribution of the antigen, after being treated with actinomycin D, suggested that this antigen is found associated with the synthesis or maturation machinery of the rRNA.

Chronic Graft-versus-Host Disease. A Model for the Study of the Autoimmune Phenomenon

C. Gelpi, Ma. A. Martinez, S. Vidal, A. Algueró, J. A. Hardin, and J. L. Rodríguez-Sanchez

Hospital de la Santa Crenu i Sant Pau, Hospital Universitari de la Facultat de Medicina de la Universitat Autónoma de Barcelona, San Antonio Ma. Claret, 167, 08025 Barcelona, Spain

Chronic graft-versus-host disease provides an experimental model for the study of the autoimmune phenomenon. In this paper we describe the clinical characteristics and serological aspects of Fl hybrid mice (Balb/c×A/J) to which spleen and lymph node cells of one or the other of the parental strains were intravenously injected.

We found that A/J cells induced the development of immunocomplex glomerulonephritis in 55% of the animals, and 25% developed inflamation of the soft parts of the upper extremities. All of the mice of this model had antinuclear antibodies, mainly antibodies to U1snRNP and anti-U3snRNP (50% and 30% respectively). Anti-DNA antibodies and anti-histone antibodies were present in 90% and 15% of the mice. The data of this study showed that this model had clinical and serological aspects of MCTD with scleroderma and SLE, with electromyographic aspects of myositis.

In contrast, Balb/c cells induced the development of vasculitis (55%); alopecia (40%); and less frequently, renal involvement. Some (50%) of the animals of this group later showed inflamation of the joints of the paws. All of the mice of this model had antinuclear antibodies. Anti-dsDNA, anti-histones and anti-snRNP antibodies were present in low titers in 50%, 25% and 35% of the animals respectively. Rheumatoid factors were the most prominent finding in the animals of this model (69%), as well as their correlation with synovitis. We conclude that this model of GVH disease shows aspects of rheumatoid arthritis and SLE.

We also describe the clinical and serological aspects induced in Fl hybrid mice (C57BL/10×DBA/2) after the intravenous injection of lymphoid cells from DBA/2 strain. In this model the prominent finding was the development of a renal disease in 65% of the animals. The antigenic specificities recognized by the antinuclear antibodies of these animals included anti-dsDNA (80%), anti-Sm (30%), anti-rRNA (70%), anti-tRNA (85%) and anti-histones (45%). Anti-histone antibodies recognized the epitopes located at the same fragments of the antigen that include the epitopes reactive with the human SLE sera. We conclude that this GVHD model had clinical and serological characteristics of active SLE, and anti-tRNA antibodies. These antibodies are frequent in human patients with polimyositis.

These studies demonstrate that the antinuclear antibodies, especially those characteristics of the human connective tissue disease, are generated during the development of a GVH disease in mice. Hence, we conclude that chronic graft versus host disease in mice provides a model for the study of the autoimmune responses that characterize human non-organ specific autoimmune diseases.

Immunogenetic Studies in Patients with Scleroderma-Associated Autoantibodies

E. Genth, R. Mierau, P. Genetzky

Rheumaklinik und Rheumaforschungsinstitut, Aachen, FRG

Patients with precipitation autoantibodies to DNA-topoisomerase I (n = 30), Pm-Scl (n = 12), or centromer-antibodies found by indirect immunofluorescent test (n = 36) were serologicaly studied for HLA class I and II antigens as well as immunoglobulin G (Gm) heavy chain and Kappa (Km) light chain allotypes. Healthy blood donors served as controls for HLA-typing (n = 85), Gm (n = 251) and Km (n = 120) testing.

Patients with anti-DNA topoisomerase I were more frequently HLA-DR5 positive (70% vs. 30.6%, p_{ex} = 0.0002, RR = 5.3) whereas HLA-DRw6 was less frequent than in controls (3.3% vs. 21.2%, p_{ex} = 0.0231, RR = 0.13). All patients with Pm-Scl-antibodies were positive for HLA-DR3 (vs. 23.5%; p_{ex} = 0.0001), and 6 patients carried the DR3/4 phenotype (50% vs. 3.5%; p_{ex} = 0.0001, RR = 27.6). Patients with centromere antibodies significantly more frequently had HLA-DR1, 4 or 8 (75% vs. 41.2%, p_{ex} = 0.0007, RR = 4.3) and less frequently HLA-DR2, 6 or 7 (19.4% vs. 69.4%, p_{ex} = 0.0001, RR = 0.11). The phenotype frequencies of immunoglobulin allotypes did not differ in patients with different scleroderma associated autoantibodies and control subjects.

We conclude the different types of scleroderma associated autoantibodies originate in association with different MHC class II antigens.

The TH Ribonucleoprotein Particle: Identity with RNase MRP and Association with RNase P

H. Gold[1], M. Bartkiewicz[2], and J. Craft[1]

[1] Yale University School of Medicine, New Haven, CT 06510, USA
[2] Polish Academy of Sciences, Warsaw, Poland

Anti-Th antibodies, first described in two patients in 1982 and thougth to be uncommon, immunoprecipitate a 7-2 RNA and an approximately 40 kilodalton polypeptide of nucleolar origin. The RNase P RNP, comprised of a 400 nucleotide RNA and unknown polypeptide(s), is an endoribonuclease that processes all precursor tRNAs to generate their mature 5' termini. We have shown previously that anti-Th antibodies immunoprecipitate H1 RNA (the RNA component of HeLa RNase P) from cell extracts (*PNAS* 85: 5483, 1988), although no structural relationship between these two RNPs has been identified.

Using immunoprecipitation of [^{32}P]labeled HeLa cell extracts, we have now identified 30 patients with anti-Th antibodies. All sera also immunoprecipitated the RNase P particle from these extracts, strongly suggesting that these two particles share an immunogenic polypeptide(s) or are structurally associated. These sera immunoprecipitated at least seven polypeptides from HeLa cell extracts labeled with [^{35}S]methionine, with a polypeptide of approximately 38 kilodaltons as a likely antigenic target.

The Th RNA from HeLa cells was sequenced and it was approximately 80% homologous with murine RNase MRP RNA, suggesting that the Th RNP and RNase MRP are identical. RNase MRP makes an endoribonucleolytic cleavage in mitochondrial primer RNA which is believed to be involved in replication of mitochondrial DNA. A sequence comparison of the Th and H1 RNAs showed that although these RNAs are distinct, they do contain some small blocks of conserved sequences which suggest a common binding site for an antigenic protein.

Of the 18 patients on whom clinical data were available, six had scleroderma (SD), five had CREST, four had isolated RAYNAUD's, two had primary biliary cirrhosis, and one had SLE with longstanding RAYNAUD's and telangiectasias. In the patients with SD, diffuse skin disease occurred in only two and renal disease in none.

These data indicate that the Th RNP and RNase MRP are the same and physically related to RNase P RNP, and in the nucleolus, the Th RNP is likely involved in RNA processing events. Like certain other autoantigenic RNPs, these particles are constituted by several polypeptides which are most likely immunoprecipitated by their linkage on an RNA backbone. Although the frequency of these antibodies is as yet unknown, they are not uncommon and they occur predominantly in patients with SD and related diseases with relatively mild clinical expression.

Immunoregulatory Effects of *Borrelia Burgdorferi* Antigens in Patients with Chronic Lyme Disease

J. J. Goronzy, L. Zöller, and C. M. Weyand

Div. of Rheum., Dept of Med., Dept. of Microbiology, University of Heidelberg, FRG

The spirochete Borrelia burgdorferi (BB) has been identified as the causative infectious agent of Lyme disease. Lyme arthritis is a rheumatic disorder which is part of a multisystemic disease attributed to a chronic persistent infection with the spirochete which is tick-transmitted. There is increasing evidence that persisting spirochetal antigen in the synovia is sustaining a chronic destructive immune response. It is unclear whether these patients fail to eliminate the infectious agent or an autoimmune response is induced by the spirochetal infection. We have studied T cell responses and requirements for antigen presentation of spirochetal antigen in patients with Lyme arthritis. Chronic borrelia infection was suspected in patients with oligoarthritic syndromes who carried IgG antibodies to BB and had no evidence of spondylarthropathy, psoriatric arthritis or rheumatoid arthritis. Interestingly, only a subgroup of patients carried circulating T lymphocytes which proliferated when stimulated with BB-pulsed syngeneic macrophages. B cells started to proliferate when incubated with ultrasonicated spirochetal antigen. B cell proliferation was dependend upon HLA-compatible T cells exluding a LPS-like mitogenic effect of the BB antigen. CD4$^+$ T cells, interleukin 2 and interleukin 4 were able to support the polyclonal B cell response induced by the spirochetal antigen. The proliferative response was inhibited in the presence of macrophages and interferon-gamma. These data sugggest that Borrelia burgdorferi includes a T-cell dependent B-cell mitogen which might substantially influence the ability of an infected host to process and to present antigen by activated B cells and might thus initiate an autoimmune reaction.

Molecular Mimicry: A Common Epitope of the (U1) snRNP Associated p68 Autoantigen and a Protein of a Human Pathogenic Virus

H. H. Guldner, H.-J. Netter, C. Szostecki, E. Jäger, and H. Will

Max-Planck-Institut für Biochemie, Am Klopferspitz 18, 8033 Martinsried, FRG

The mechanisms leading to autoimmunity are not known but one possible concept is crossreaction of antibodies with epitopes shared by microbial antigens and host self-components referred to as molecular mimicry. A self-antigen target for anti-(U1)snRNP autoantibodies which are characteristic for certain inflammatory rheumatic diseases is a particle-associated 68 kDa protein (p68). The corresponding gene has been cloned and three major autoantigenic domains have been identified. One of the antigenic domains (domain A) shows sequence similarity to group specific nucleocapsid proteins (gag-protein) of animal retroviruses and this led to the speculation that similar human viruses play a role in initiation of p68 autoimmune response.

To investigate the significance of this sequence similarity with retroviral sequences, to determine whether there is more than one epitope in this region, and to identify the amino acids involved in autoantibody binding, detailed epitope mapping and search for shared epitopes with other sequences have been performed.

Wildtype and mutant domain A polypeptide sequences expressed as fusion proteins in *E. coli* or synthetic peptides derived from domain A were used as substrates in immunoblotting and ELISA assays. According to the reaction patterns of a collection of anti-p68 autoantibody positive sera three groups of sera were identified: group I contained antibodies binding to a sequence 20 amino acids long which presumably represents a discontinuous epitope; group II sera reacted with a five amino acid motif and group III sera contained both of these antibody specificities. The 5 amino acid sequence motif was also found on a protein of a highly prevalent human pathogenic virus. Crossreaction of the p68 autoantibody with the 5 amino acid sequence motif in the viral sequence context could be demonstrated with antibodies affinity purified from domain A containing fusion proteins. The common epitope recognized by antibodies of autoimmune sera suggests that these human viruses may play a role in initiation of autoimmunity to the well-known p68 antigen. This working hypothesis is currently under investigation.

Human Autoantibodies to Synaptonemal Complex

T. Haaf, A. Machens, and M. Schmid

Department of Human Genetics, University of Würzburg, Würzburg, FRG

Autoantibodies to synaptonemal complex (SC) are spontaneously produced by patients with various autoimmune diseases. The synaptonemal complex forms the proteinaceous axis between pairing chromosomes during meiotic prophase;

SC formation appears to be an essential prerequisite for chromosome pairing, recombination and homologue disjunction.

Immunofluorescent staining of pachytene cells localized the autoantigen to the central element or the transverse filaments of the SC but not to the lateral elements. In leptotene and zygotene spermatocytes, antigenic SC structures are not at all detectable. The earliest stage of meiotic prophase which contains the SC antigen is pachytene. At higher magnification, the antigenic SC structure shows a relatively uniform longitudinal segmentation. The SC ends which are known to attach to the nuclear envelope are characterized by a thickened segment of variable size. The longitudinal segmentation of the SCs does not correspond to the chromomere pattern of pachytene bivalents; most probably, it reflects a structural or functional property of the SCs themselves. Specific antibody labeling is confined to the SC at synapsis. The lateral elements of unpaired homologues at leptotene and zygotene as well as the unpaired axes of the X and Y chromosomes during pachytene are not labeled. The antigenic SC structure is definitely lost during diplotene. Therefore, it can be hypothesized that the SC antigen is involved in stage-specific processes such as chromosome pairing and recombination.

Cytochemical tests revealed the SC antigen to be a hydrophobic non-histone protein bound to DNA. It cannot be extracted by balanced salt solutions, high ionic strength solutions and non-ionic detergents. The nature of the SC antigen and its insolubility are reminiscent of the biochemical composition of the nuclear skeleton and the mitotic chromosome scaffold, respectively.

An unusual characteristic of the SC autoantigen is its species specificity. Patients were found whose sera selectively labeled the SCs of human, mouse or newts. Nevertheless, most anti-SC antisera demonstrate minor cross-reactions between different pachytene cell substrates indicating that the SCs share some ubiquitous antigenic components.

Immunolocalization and Number of Transcriptionally Active rRNA Genes in Vertebrate Cells

T. Haaf and M. Schmid

Department of Human Genetics, University of Würzburg, Würzburg, FRG

Under the action of the adenosine analogue DRB, the normally compact nucleoli are spread through the nuclear interior forming several beaded strands.

The maximum number of nucleolar necklaces (NN) corresponds to the number of nucleolus organizing chromosomes. The tandemly arranged granules of these NN then reflect the linear distribution of rRNA genes along the nucleolus organizer regions. The granules stain silver (Ag)-positive and bind human autoantibodies to RNA polymerase I (RPI), both properties thought to be characteristic for an active rDNA conformation. Each granule represents an individual transcription unit consisting of an 18S + 28S rRNA gene and the transcriptional machinery. Adjacent granules are separated by nontranscribed spacer regions.

The number of RPI-positive granules and, thus, of transcriptionally active rRNA genes was determined in fibroblast cells of the following vertebrate species:

Species	Number of transcription units	Number of chromosomal NORs
Human	115	8
Cavia cobaya	145	10
Mus musculus	106	6
Sminthopsis crassicaudata	59	2
Macropus eugenii (female)	72	2
Macropus eugenii (male)	45	1
Gallus domesticus	61	2
Bufo rubropunctatus	70	2
Gastrotheca riobambae (female)	80	2
Gastrotheca riobambae (male)	51	1

Mammals whose karyotypes are endowed with multiple NORs also exhibit a higher number of transcriptionally active rRNA genes per diploid genome than marsupials and lower vertebrates. Correspondingly, species with X-linked NORs show sex specific differences in the number of transcription units.

Mouse pachytene spermatocytes contain 54 RPI-positive granules on the average, round spermatids 33. Compared to somatic fibroblasts, only a percentage of rRNA genes is transcriptionally active during meiosis and spermiogenesis.

Mapping of Autoimmune Reactive Sites on snRNP Proteins

W. J. Habets

Department of Biochemistry, University of Nijmegen, P.O. Box 9101, 6500 HB Nijmegen, The Netherlands

Antibodies from patients with SLE react with snRNP particles and inhibit pre-mRNA splicing *in vitro*. Therefore it is thought that these autoantibodies recognize functional sites on snRNA-associated proteins. For this reason, but also because knowledge of the primary structure of autoimmune epitopes might provide insight in the etiology of autoimmune diseases, we undertook epitope mapping experiments with the U1 snRNP-specific A protein and the U2 snRNP-specific B″ protein.

Random DNAse I fragments of cDNA clones encoding these two closely related proteins (ref. 1 and 2) were expressed in λgt11 and recombinant plaques were screened with antibodies from an SLE patient. Two antigenic sites were mapped on the A protein which we termed epitope 1 and epitope 2 (ref. 3). Epitope 1 (PPPGMIPPPGLAPGQIPPGAM) is situated in a proline-rich region of the A protein that has no counterpart on the B″ protein. When this proline-rich region was compared with the primary structure of other snRNP proteins, however, epitope 1-like regions were found in snRNA-associated proteins B′, B, C and N. Screening of a larg number of patients sera revealed that the epitope 1-like regions on all these snRNP proteins were targeted by specific subsets of autoantibodies. Epitope 1-reactive antibodies could be affinity purified from anti-Sm and anti-U(U1, U2)RNP sera and were shown to cross-react with either snRNP proteins B′/B, N and an as yet unidentified 50K non-snRNP protein, or with snRNP proteins B′/B and C. To substantiate these findings, we synthesized peptides based on the epitope 1 region of protein A and the epitope 1-like region of protein N. These peptides reacted in ELISA with antibodies from SLE sera. Epitope 2 (PGFKEVRLVPGRHDIAFVEFDNEVQ) is situated in a region of the A protein that is highly similar to a carboxy terminal region in protein B″. It was therefore not surprising that epitope 2 bound A and B″ cross-reactive antibodies from anti-(U1, U2)RNP patients sera. Epitope 2-reactive antibodies were not found in anti-Sm or anti-(U1)RNP sera.

Using a deletion mutagenesis approach, at least three other autoepitopecontaining regions on the A protein could be identified. One of these regions contained an immunodominant epitope reactive with a least 70% of anti-snRNP sera from patients with different connective tissue diseases.

For the mapping of epitopes on the U2 snRNP-specific B″ protein we used monoclonal anti-U2 RNP antibodies obtained from Balb/c mice immunized with recombinant β-galactosidase-B″ fusion protein. Two monoclonal antibodies (mAbs) appeared to cross-react with proteins A and B″ (and thus with U1 and U2 snRNPs) whereas one exclusivley recognized protein B″ (and consequently reacted only with U2 snRNPs). Epitope mapping employing a DNase I fragment library of the B″ cDNA showed that the three mAb-reactive regions were discontinuous and that they substantially overlapped. All three mAb-reactive epitopes comprised the epitope 2 analogue of protein B″. Competition experiments with anti-(U1, U2)RNP patients sera showed that all three monoclonal antibodies defined autoimmune reactive sites.

From the above findings it is concluded that the anti-snRNP immune response in patients with connective tissue diseases is polyclonal and most probably antigen-driven.

References

1. HABETS, W. J., SILLEKENS, P. T. G., HOET, M. H., SCHALKEN, J. A., ROEBROEK, A. J. M. LEUNISSEN, J. A. M., VAN DE VEN, W. J. M., VAN VENROOIJ, W. J. (1987): Analysis of a cDNA clone expressing a human autoimmune antigen: full-lenght sequence of the U2 small nuclear RNA-associated B″ antigen. Proc. Natl. Acad. Sci. USA **84**, 2421–2425
2. SILLEKENS, P. T. G., HABETS, W. J. A., BEIJER R. P., VAN VENROOIJ, W. J. (1987): cDNA cloning of the human U1 snRNA associated A protein: Extensive homology between U1 and U2 snRNP specific proteins. EMBO J. **6**, 3841–3848
3. HABETS, W. J., SILLEKENS, P. T. G., HOET, M. H., McALLISTER, G., LERNER, M. R., VAN VENROOIJ, W. J.: B cell autoepitopes of the human U1 snRNP-specific A protein are immunologically conserved in small nuclear ribonucleoproteins. Proc. Natl. Acad. Sci. USA in press

Clinical Significances of Rare Autoantibodies to Small Nuclear and Cytoplasmic Ribonucleoproteins

N. Hama, T. Mimori, M. Akizuki, and M. Homma

Keio University School of Medicine, Tokyo, Japan

This study attempts to clarify the clinical significances of infrequent autoantibodies reactive with small nuclear and cytoplasmic ribonucleoproteins.

405 sera from patients with connective tissue diseases were screened by protein A-facilitated immunoprecipitation (LERNER-STEITZ assay) using ^{32}P-labeled HeLa cell extracts as antigen sources. Immunoprecipitated RNAs were frac-

tionated on urea-PAGE and detected by autoradiography. The results of our study are summarized in the table.

Table: Frequencies of autoantibodies to ribonucleoproteins

Antibodies to: (precipitated RNA)		SLE (126) (%)	PSS (113) (%)	PM/DM (51) (%)	Overlap (115) (%)
U1RNP	(U1RNA)	21	12	4	46
Ro/SS-A	(Y1-Y5RNA)	42	20	10	34
La/SS-B	(La-RNA)	17	7	2	10
Sm	(U1, U2, U4-sRNA)	29	4	0	29
Ribosome	(rRNA)	4	1	2	1
U3RNP	(U3RNA)	1	7	0	1
7-2RNP	(7-2RNA)	1	4	0	1
Jo-1	(tRNA^{his})	0	0	29	3
PL-7	(tRNA^{thr})	0	0	4	1
PL-12	(tRNA^{ala})	0	0	2	0
SRP	(7SL-RNA)	0	0	6	0
U1/U2R-NP	(U1/U2RNA)	0	0	0	9

Anti-U3RNP and anti-7-2RNP antibodies defined among sera containing anti-nucleolar reactivity in immunofluorescence appeared to be specific markers for PSS. Anti-U3RNP antibodies were associated with PSS characterized by a low prevalence of lung involvement. Anti-7-2RNP antibodies were detected in patients with limited form of scleroderma. Antibodies to aminoacyl-tRNA synthetases (Jo-1, PL-7 and PL-12) were strongly associated with PM/DM with chronic interstitial lung disease characterized by "shrinking lung" and polyarthritis. Anti-SRP (Signal Recognition Particle) antibodies were detected specifically in patients with intractable PM/DM. Antibodies which precipitated selectively U1 and U2RNa (anti-U1/U2RNP) were identified in sera with anti-U1RNP only by immunodiffuison, and strongly associated with overlap syndrome characterized by scleroderma and inflammatory myositis.

Detailed analysis of the fine specificities of autoantibodies reactive with RNPs disclosed the presence of unique patient groups which were not identified by the conventional immunological methods.

Molecular Cloning and Expression of cDNAs Encoding snRNP Polypeptide Autoantigens

S. O. Hoch, J. A. Haselby, M. Jannatipour, and L. A. Rokeach

The Agouron Institute, La Jolla, CA 92037, USA

Anti-Sm is an antibody specificity associated with the autoimmune disease systemic lupus erythematosus. Sm antibodies precipitate the small nuclear ribonucleoprotein (SnRNP) complexes which contain the U1, U2, U4, U5 and U6 snRNAs and a minimum of eleven polypetides. Functionally the Sm snRNP are involved in the maturation of the nascent mRNA transcript. Each snRNP contains a common *core* of six polypeptides of which three, the B' (27 000 molecular weight), B (26 000 m.w.) and D (13 000 m.w.) proteins, are synonymous with the major Sm autoantigens. The Sm snRNP have proven readily amenable to isolation. Once isolated, the snRNP are resistant to chromatographic fractionation into the individual polypeptides; however, there are compelling reasons to have such moieties relative to these proteins as snRNP components and as autoantigens. Thus, we undertook to circumvent this problem by cloning the cDNAs encoding the three Sm polypeptides of interest, B', B and D. Amino-terminal sequences were obtained for the three polypeptides. These sequences were used to design oligonucleotide probes to successfully screen a human B-lymphocyte cDNA library for clones encoding Sm-D (1) and Sm-B'/B (2). Evaluation of the predicted amino acid sequences suggested the importance of the carboxy-terminal sequence of both Sm-D and Sm-B'/B relative to their immunoreactivity and function as snRNP components. In order to study these features we have undertaken the heterologous expression of these Sm autoantigens in different prokaryotic and eukaryotic hosts. Sm-B'/B was expressed in an immunoreactive form as a fusion protein with TrpE (anthranilate synthase) of *E. coli*. Multiple translational fusions between this bacterial *trpE* gene and fragments encompassing the length of the Sm-B'/B coding sequence were constructed. All were screened by immunoblotting against a number of autoimmune sera. These analyses showed that the major Sm determinant was located at the carboxyterminus of the protein, in the region containing a proline-rich repetitive unit that is shared with other snRNP and nucleic acid binding proteins. The same approach, using TrpE fusion, has been utilized for Sm-D epitope mapping, underscoring the importance of the glycine-arginine repeated motif at its carboxy terminus. Experiments continue to allow for the expression of these polypeptides in different host systems to study the possible effect of posttranslational modification on immunoreactivity and to generate non-fusion entities to facilitate analyses of the assembly of the *core* snRNA structure.

Our investigations also extend to the class of snRNP which are associated with the Ro and La antigens that are characteristic of the disease Sjögren's syndrome. Particular emphasis has been placed on the Ro antigen. Ro is present in the cell as part of an RNP complex whose RNA components are designated Y RNAs. Despite the cytoplasmic localization of the Y RNAs and, therefore, by inference of the Ro protein, there is conflicting data suggesting both nuclear and cytoplasmic localization for Ro. The actual function of the Ro RNP remains obscure; possible involvement in translation and in mRNA transport and storage has been hypothesized. With the aim to determine the molecular structure of the Ro polypeptide(s), we decided to clone the cDNA encoding at least one of the Ro antigens. The approach was the same as for the Sm antigens, but in this case we designed an oligonucleotide probe based on a published-amino-terminal sequences for a 60000 m.w. Ro species (3). Positive clones were identified and sequenced. One such clone, designated 38-1, has a codon composition exactly matching that of the published Ro sequence. In addition, analysis of the deduced sequence with that of the mature protein reveals the presence of a putative 17-amino acid long signal peptide with a canonical alanine residue at its proposed processing site. This raises interesting questions regarding the function and compartmentalization of Ro. The carboxy-terminal part of the predicted Ro amino acid sequence is very rich in charged residues, particularly acidic ones, which may have relevance to Ro as an autoantigen.

References

1. ROKEACH, L. A., HASELBY, J. A., HOCH, S. O. (1988): Proc. Natl. Acad. Sci. USA **85**, 4832
2. ROKEACH, L. A., JANNATIPOUR, M., HASELBY, J. A., HOCH, S. O. (1989): J. Biol. Chem. **264**, 5024
3. LIEU, T.-S., NEWKIRK, M. M., CAPRA, J. D., SONTHEIMER, R. D. (1988): J. Clin. Invest. **82**, 96

U1-68Kd Protein-Positive Mixed Connective Tissue Disease is Associated with HLA-DR4 and Appears Genetically Distinct from Systemic Lupus Erythematosus

R. W. Hoffman, L. J. Rettenmaier, Y. Takeda, and G. C. Sharp

University of Missouri-Columbia and the Harry S. Truman Veterans Hospital Columbia, MO 65201, USA

Mixed connective tissue disease (MCTD) and systemic lupus erythematosus (SLE) are two prototype multi-systemic autoimmune diseases of unknown etiology. These two diseases are characterized by distinct clinical features and the presence of distinct patterns of autoantibodies which are reactive with selfantigens, including autoantibodies reactive with small nuclear ribonucleoproteins (snRNPs). The existence of MCTD as a distinct disease entity is, however, controversial. Some investigators consider MCTD to be a subset of SLE while others include it within the spectrum of scleroderma.

To investigate whether MCTD is a distinct entity we studied 20 North American Caucasian MCTD patients whose sera were reactive with the U1-68Kd protein antigen of the snRNP complex by an enzyme-linked immunoabsorbent assay (ELISA), using the purified 68Kd protein antigen or a recombinant fusion protein for the antigen. Sera from all 20 MCTD patients studied were positive for reactivity with the 68Kd protein antigen; 12 of 38 SLE patients sera were positive for reactivity with the B/B′ and D proteins (the Sm antigen) of the snRNP complex. We compared the MCTD patients to 38 SLE patients and normal controls.

All patients classified as MCTD had typical overlapping clinical features and met the classification criteria of Porter, et al. (Arthritis Rheum. 1989: 31, 219); all patients classified as SLE met 4 or more of the revised American Rheumatism Association criteria for SLE. All patients were all examined using the snRNP ELISA assay to determine whether their sera reacted with the 68Kd, A, B/B, or D proteins or the snRNP complex. HLA-A, B, C typings were performed using standard the NIH complement-dependent cytotoxicity technique. HLA-DR and HLA-DQ typing were performed using a two-color fluorescence technique.

Results are shown below. HLA-DR4 was increased in MCTD (60%) versus (30%) controls ($P < 0.02$) and versus (18%) SLE ($P < 0.002$). The supratypic HLA marker HLA-DRw53 was increased in (80%) MCTD patients versus (53%) controls ($P < 0.008$) and versus (37%) SLE ($P < 0.004$). The supratypic HLA marker HLA-DRw52 was increased in SLE (76%) versus (30%) MCTD ($P < 0.004$). HLA-DR3 was increased in SLE (47%) versus (21%) controls $P < 0.004$. HLA-DR2 was increased in MCTD (50%) and SLE (53%) versus controls (27%) $P < 0.002$.

Table: HLA-DR and DQ typing results

HLA Antigen	Percent				
	68KD+MCTD n = 20	ALL SLE n = 38	Sm+SLE n = 12	Sm−SLE n = 26	Controls n = 102
DRW52	30[1]	76	78	75	65
DRW53	80[2]	37	33	38	53
DR1	20	8	8	8	16
DR2	50	53[5]	75	42	27
DR3	15[3]	47[6]	42	58	21
DR4	60[4]	18	25	15	30
DR5	0	13	17	12	30
DQW1	65	74	75	73	67
DQW2	45	58	50	62	35
DQW3	65	37	50	62	60

[1] $p < 0.008$ MCTD versus control; $p < 0.004$ MCTD versus SLE.
[2] $p < 0.02$ MCTD versus control; $p < 0.002$ MCTD versus SLE.
[3] $p < 0.01$ MCTD versus SLE.
[4] $p < 0.002$ MCTD versus SLE; $p < 0.02$ MCTD versus controls.
[5] $p < 0.002$ SLE versus controls.
[6] $p < 0.004$ SLE versus controls.

We found no significant differences between the distribution of phenotypes for any HLA-A, B or C antigen tested between MCTD of SLE patients and controls.

Thus, MCTD patients with elevated levels of autoantibody reactive with the 68 Kd protein of the snRNP complex had disease associated with HLA-DR4, SLE patients without reactivity against the 68Kd or Sm protein antigens of the snRNP complex had disease associated with HLA-DR3 and HLA-DR2; while Sm positive SLE patients with elevated level of autoantibody reactive with the B/B′ and D (Sm) proteins of the snRNP complex had disease associated with HLA-DR2 and HLA-DR3, but not HLA-DR4.

Our study is the first to examine HLA antigen frequencies in a North American Caucasian U1-68 Kd protein-positive MCTD patient population. This study is unique in that we have examined a group of ethnically homogenous patients with specifically defined clinical and serological characteristics. The selection of patients with MCTD and reactivity with the U1-68 Kd protein using the protein specific ELISA, and comparison of this group with an ethnically and geographically matched group of U1-68 Kd protein-negative SLE patients and healthy controls provides the opportunity to examine the influence of HLA-linked genetic difference on these two related diseases. From this study we have confirmed and extended the observations of others and shown that the HLA-DR4 phenotype is increased in North American Caucasian patients with MCTD. This HLA-DR4 linked genetic susceptibility to U1-68 Kd protein-positive MCTD appears to be distinct from the association of SLE with HLA-DR3, which was found in our local SLE group and as has been reported in many other studies on SLE. Also of interest from this study is the fact that we found no association of U1-68 Kd positive MCTD with any of the HLA antigens previously reported to be associated with scleroderma, including HLA-A9, B8, DR3 and DR5.

We conclude that U1-68 Kd protein-positive MCTD appears to be most strongly associated with HLA-DR4 and/or haplotypes bearing the supratypic marker HLA-DRw53. U1-68 Kd protein-positive MCTD appears genetically distinct from SLE which is associated with HLA-DR3 and HLA-DR2.

A Novel Trait of Naturally-Occurring Anti-DNA Antibodies: Dissociation from Immune Complexes in Neutral 0.3 – 0.5 M NaCl

Y. Kanai[1], T. Kubota[2]

[1] Department of Molecular Oncology, Institute of Medical Science, University of Tokyo, Japan
[2] First Department of Internal Medicine, Tokyo Medical and Dental University, Tokyo, Japan

Monoclonal and polyclonal anti-DNA antibodies from autoimmune mice, and experimentally-induced rabbit anti-nucleic acid polyclonal antibodies were tested for stability of binding to nucleic acids in the presence of various concentrations of NaCl by an enzyme-linked immunosorbent assay (ELISA). Murine monoclonal antibodies 2ClO (IgG2b) and lA2 (IgG2a), which are known to react specifically with double-stranded(ds) DNA, dissociated completely from their complexes with DNA when washed with neutral 0.5 M NaCl solution. Another monoclonal antibody (MoAb) (IgM, K), which is polyreactive with singlestranded(ss) DNA, cardiolipin, and trinitrophenyl hapten (TNP), was also dissociated from its complexes with ssDNA, but not from its complexes with TNP, by 0.3 – 0.5 M NaCl. Similar differencies were observed in the stabilities of bindings of serum antibodies from autommune mice to DNA and TNP. In contrast anti-nucleic acid polyclonal antibodies induced in rabbits by immunization with poly(I), poly(dT) or poly(ADP-ribose) were not significantly dissociated from their immune complexes with relevant antigens or DNA by 0.5 M NaCl. The finding that nucleic acid antigens were not detached from a solid phase by washing with 0.5 M NaCl solution indicated that the reductions of binding of anti-DNA antibodies in both MoAbs and naturally-occurring antibodies were really due to dissociation of the antibodies from immune complexes. This is the first demonstration that DNA epitopes recognized by naturally-occurring antibodies in both systemic lupus erythematosus (SLE) and its model mice are sensitive to neutral NaCl concentrations. This novel trait of naturally-occurring antibodies will be very useful in studies on the nature of immune complexes in the sera and kidney of cases of SLE.

Immunoblotting Analysis in Antigenic Components of Circulating Immune Complexes of Rheumatoid Arthritis and Systemic Lupus Erythematosus Patients

R. Kasukawa, Y. Sato, Y. Okubo, and T. Nishimaki

Second Department of Internal Medicine, Fukushima Medical College, Fukushima, Japan

In order to analyze the antigenic components in circulating immune complexes (IC) in patients with rheumatoid arthritis (RA) and systemic lupus erythematosus (SLE), immune complexes in serum or joint fluid (JF) were isolated in using solid phase Clq tubes and analyzed for their components through immunoblotting method.

In separation of RA IC on SPS-PAGE, components of 73, 54 and 27 kD bands were identified as μ chain of IgM, γ chain of IgG, and L chain of Ig respectively. These components were transfered to cellulose acetate membrane and allowed to react with IgM fraction of RA serum or RA JF obtained through Sephadex G-200 filtration under acid condition. The IgM fraction could react with 54 kD (γ chain of IgG) component but not with other components.

Five SLE IC samples taken from 5 patients who have anti-DNA antibody commonly besides other antibodies were tested on the cellulose acetate membrane against HeLa extract separated on SDS-PAGE. Several bands were demonstrated on the membrane by the anti-human IgG antibody with mobilities ranging from 76 to 16 kD. However, in the reaction between the purified plasmid DNA separated on SDS-PAGE and SLE IC in serum, only 16 kD band was identified by the anti-human IgG antibody.

The DNA in SLE IC was labelled by ^{32}P through multiprime labelling method and separated on SDS-PAGE. The autoradiography showed wide bands with mobilities ranging from 300 to 50 base pairs. The dot hybridization test for binding of ^{32}P labelled DNA in SLE IC to DNA from various species showed a binding to autologous DNA in IC and DNA taken from human hepatoma and HeLa cells but not from E. coli, salmon nor calf thymus.

From these results, we could find IgG in RA IC and DNA of human origin in SLE IC as one of their antigenic components.

The Human La Autoantigen Contains an RNA Binding Domain and an ATP Binding Domain

D. J. Kenan and J. D. Keene

Department of Microbiology and Immunology, Duke University Medical Center, Durham, NC 27710, USA

Some rheumatologic disorders such as systemic lupus erythematosus and SJÖGREN's syndrome are characterized by the formation of autoantibodies reactive with the La antigen. Biochemical analysis of the La antigen in a wide variety of vertebrate cells has shown it to be a ribunucleprotein (RNP) complex consisting of a 48 000 Dalton phosphoprotein, termed La, associated with any of the precursor transcripts produced by RNA polymerase III, including pre-tRNA and pre-5S RNA. GOTTLIEB and STEITZ (EMBO J. **8**, 841 – 861, 1989) have demonstrated that La protein associates with RNA polymerase III transcription complexes and that termination of transcription is impaired in the absence of La.

The human La cDNA was cloned using La-specific patient serum as a probe (CHAMBERS et al., J. Biol. Chem. **263**:18 043 – 18 051, 1988), and the cDNA was expressed in several prokaryotic systems and in rabbit reticulocyte lysates. cDNA-encoded protein produced in these systems retained RNA binding specificity identical to that of HeLa La protein as assayed by RNP immunoprecipitation and by gel shift analysis. A 76 amino acid sequence was noted in the second quarter of the La protein sequence that matched the consensus RNA recognition motif (RRM) as defined by QUERY et al. (Cell **57**:89 – 101, 1989). A 131 residue truncated La protein, produced in E. coli and containing the RRM, retained the ability to interact with precursor RNA polymerase III transcripts. These findings are consistent with the hypothesis that the RRM constitutes part of an RNA binding domain in La as well as in other RRM proteins.

Near the C-terminus of the conceptual La protein sequence are found two tandem consensus ATP binding motifs. UV crosslinking experiments using La protein overproduced in *E. coli* showed that La bound to ATP. A proteolytic peptide of HeLa La protein representing the C-terminal 185 residues, including the two ATP binding motifs, was shown by CHAN and TAN (Mol. Cell. Biol. 7:2588−2591, 1987) to contain all of the phosphorylated residues of La protein. Two dimensional gel analysis revealed four or five charge isomers of La protein related to phosphorylation and/or ATP binding.

These results suggest that the La protein has two structural domains: an N-terminal RNA binding domain and a C-terminal ATP binding domain that is phosphorylated. Secondary structure predictions suggest that much of La is α-helical, including an exceptionally long putative helix stabilized by numerous salt bridges that connects the RNA binding domain to the ATP binding domain. A role for phosphorylation of La protein has not been determined, although possible functions include the regulation of protein-RNA interactions in La RNPs as well as protein-protein interactions in RNA polymerase III transcription complexes. We are currently investigating the amino acid sequences responsible for conferring specificity to La protein-RNA interactions and the role of RNA binding in La-dependent transcription termination by RNA polymerase III.

Autoantibodies to "HSP 70 Class" Proteins in Sera of Systemic Lupus Erythematosus (SLE) Patients and Healthy Subjects. A Spontaneous Expression of HSP 70 Autoantibodies

I. Kindas-Mügge and I. Fröhlich

Institute of Tumor Biology and Cancer Research, University of Vienna, Vienna, Italy

Systemic lupus erythematosus (SLE) is a prototypic autoimmune disease containing autoantibodies to various small nuclear and cytoplasmic ribonucleoprotein complexes. These antibodies serve as markers of diagnostic and prognostic significance.

It was recently found that an enhancement of heat shock protein (hsp) synthesis occur in peripheral blood mononuclear cells from SLE patients [1]. Although the precise function of hsp(s) is not yet fully understood, their presumed role is to protect cells from injury. Since there has been no information about autoantibodies to heat shock proteins, we decided to look for sera containing autoantibodies to the mammalian "hsp 70 class" proteins, one of the most prominent class of heat shock proteins.

In the following study "hsp 70 class" proteins were isolated from Ht-1080 cells by a modification of the method reported by WELCH et al. [2]. The heat "inducible" hsp 72 kDa protein as well as the "constitutive" hsp 73 kDa protein were used as antigen source in immunoblotting experiments. In some experiments a protein of 75 kDa, copurifying with the hsp 70 group proteins and known as non inducible protein with great sequence homology to the hsp 70 s [2] was included as antigen source. Sera obtained from SLE patients were analyzed for antibodies against the isolated heat shock proteins. The antibodies of some sera showed reactivity towards the proteins with molecular weight of 72 000 and 73 000. The 75 000 copurifying heat shock protein was also recognized by some sera. However, sera from normal subjects, tested for their reaction to a hsp 70 protein extract showed surprisingly similar reactivity to the respective proteins as sera from SLE patients. No significant difference was noted between the two groups of individuals tested.

In the study herein, we demonstrate that autoantibodies, found in sera from SLE patients as well as in healthy subjects, recognize the "hsp 70 class" proteins. These findings indicate the possibility that hsp 70 s can serve as in vivo immunogens, capable of inducing a spontaneous expression of autoantibodies.

References

1. DEGUCHI, I. Y. (1987): Biochem. Biophys. Res. Commun. **148, 3**, 1063
2. WELCH, W. J. (1985): Mol. Cell. Biol. **5, 6**, 1229

Cross-Reactive Rheumatoid Factor in Rheumatoid Arthritis with Extra-Articular Disease

M. Kinoshita, S. Aotsuka, and R. Yokohari

Division of Immunology, Clinical Research Institute, National Medical Center, Tokyo, Japan

Rheumatoid factors (RF) have been shown to have considerable heterogeneity and bind not only with IgG but also with a variety of substances, such as nuclear histone, nitrophenyl groups or single-stranded DNA (ssDNA).

In the present study, we investigated the appearance of IgM, RF cross-reactive with ssDNA in sera from patients with rheumatoid arthritis (RA), SJOGREN's syndrome, systemic lupus erythematosus and progressive systemic sclerosis.

Titers of IgM RF and IgM antibodies to ssDNA were measured using an ELISA procedure. Isolation of RF was carried out by incubation of serum with human IgG-coupled Sepharose followed by elution with sodium acetate buffer (pH 4.0).

The study disclosed that polyclonal RF cross-reactive with ss-DNA (CRRF) are widely distributed in a variety of rheumatic diseases, and that their serum level is significantly high in RA with extra-articular disease (EARA). CRRF would be a useful marker for a clinical subset of RA. High prevalence rate of CRRF in EARA may suggest its pathogenetic role in the extra-particular manifestation of the disease, although the precise mechanism is not clear.

Profiles of Anti-Nuclear Antibodies in Scleroderma Spectrum Disorders

H. Kondo, N. Takashina, and S. Kashiwazaki

Department of Internal Medicine, Kitasato University School of Medicine, Japan

In 112 scleroderma patients which satisfied the criteria for systemic sclerosis of ARA and 43 patients with sclerodactyly and RAYNAUD's phenomenon (SR), anti-nuclear antibodies were studied. The presence of anti-centromere antibody (ACA) was detected by staining of centromeres of chromosomes from Wi12 cells. A nuclear enriched sonicate of HeLa cell proteins was prepared for immunoblotting as described by MCNEILAGE et al. to investigate antibodies to U1-RNP, Scl-70 and centromeric antigens. Furthermore, 17 kD centromeric antigen was purified by immunoaffinity chromatography from the prepared crude antigens. Immunoblotting was also performed using the purified 17 kD antigen.

Anti-nuclear antibody was detected by immunofluorescence using HEp-2 cell in 95 of the 112 patients with scleroderma and in 36 of 43 with SR. Anti-Scl-70 antibody was detected in 32 of scleoderma sera and none of SR by immunodiffusion. Thirty-one of 32 anti-Scl-70 antibody positive sera showed antibody for 95 kD protein by immunoblotting. Twenty-eight of scleroderma and 18 of SR had precipitating antibodies to U1-RNP. Twenty-six of 28 positive sera from scleroderma and 13 of 18 positive sera from SR reacted with the 68 kD U1-RNP associated protein. Six of 7 sera which did not react with 68 kD protein recognized other U1-RNP associated proteins. Three patients (2.5%) with scleroderma had both anti-Scl-70 and anti-U1-RNP antibodies. ACA was detected in 17 of scleroderma and 18 of SR by immunofluorescence. Antibody to 17 kD protein was demonstrated in 34 of 35 ACA positive sera by immunoblotting using the crude antigen. All of the 34 sera reacted with 17 kD protein purified by the immunoaffinity chromatography. Two patients with SR had both ACA and anti-U1-RNP antibody. These sera reacted with 68 kD, A and 17 kD protein. One patient with scleroderma had ACA and anti-Scl-70 antibody.

These studies showed that the predominant ANA in scleroderma was anti-Scl-70 antibody and the main ANA in SR were ACA and anti-U1-RNP antibodies. Furthermore, immunoblotting using crude antigens and purified 17 kD centomeric antigen was useful for detection of two different system antibodies including ACA and anti-ENA antibody.

Desmin Antibodies in Acute Myopericarditis

P. Kurki, J. Karjalainen, A. Hautanen, and I. Virtanen

Dept. of Bacteriology and Immunology, Dept. of Anatomy, University of Helsinki, First Dept. of Medicine, Helsinki University Central Hospital, and Central Military Hospital I, Helsinki, Finland

The role of autoantibodies against cardiac tissue in the pathogenesis of acute (infectious) myopericarditis is poorly understood − partly because the specificity of the antibodies is unknown (WOODROFF, 1980). We assay circulating antibodies against desmin, the main component of intermediate filaments of muscle cells (LAZARIDES, 1982), in 18 patients with acute infectious myopericarditis (AM), in ten patients with acute myocardial infarction, in 24 patients with acute uncomplicated infections, and in 68 blood donors by an enzyme-linked immunosorbent assay using purified desmin from PURKINJE fibers of cow heart as antigen. In addition, anti-heart antibodies were assayed by indirect immunofluorescence using rat heart as the target.

Anti-heart antibodies were detected in all patient groups: Antibodies reacting with arterial smooth muscle were detected in 67% of patients with acute myocarditis (AM), 70% of patients with myocardial infarction (MI), and in 16% of patients with acute uncomplicated infections (AI). Antibodies giving a striational staining pattern of muscle fibers were seen in 39%, 10%, and 48% of patients with AM, MI, and AI, respectively.

The cut off point for the anti-desmin assay were set at the mean + 2 SD of the blood donors values. The results are seen in Table 1.

Table 1. Desmin antibodies in patient sera

Diagnosis	Anti-Desmin		
	IgG	IgM	Total
Myopericarditis	3/18 (17%)	4/18 (22%)	7/18 (39%)
Myocardial infarction	0/10	0/10	0/10
Acute infection	0/24	1/24 (4%)	1/24 (4%)

All anti-desmin-positive patients with myopericarditis had also anti-heart antibodies by indirect immunofluorescence. Serial samples were available from two anti-desmin-positive patients with myopericarditis. In both cases the level on anti-desmin decreased upon recovery.

The role of cytoskeleton as a target for autoantibodies is well known (KURKI and VIRTANEN, 1984). Autoantibodies to the cytoskeleton of heart cells have been reported previously in patients with pericarditis (MAISCH et al., 1982; NICHOLSON et al., 1977). Our results show that muscle-specific autoantibodies are associated with acute (infectious) myopericarditis. In addition, the use of a purified antigen in a quantitative assay seems to offer better diagnostic specificity and an opportunity to follow up an immunoglobulin class-specific autoantibody response.

References

KURKI, P., VIRTANEN, I. (1984): The detection of human antibodies against cytoskeletal components. J. Immunol. Methods. **76**, 329

LAZARIDES, E. (1982): Intermediate filaments: A chemically heterogenous developmentally regulated class of proteins. Annu. Rev. Biochem. **51**, 219

MAISCH, B., MAISCH, S., KOCHSIEK, K. (1982): Immune reactions in tuberculous and chronic constrictive pericarditis. Am. J. Cardiol. **50**, 1007

NICHOLSON, G., DAWKINS, R., MCDONALD, R., WETHERALL, J. (1977): A classification of heart antibodies: Differentiation between heart-specific and heterophile antibodies. Clin. Immunol. Immunopathol. **7**, 349

WOODROFF, J. (1980): Viral myocarditis. A review. Am. J. Pathol. **101**, 427

Ankylosing Spondylitis (AS) and Rheumatoid Arthritis (RA): Improved Diagnosis and Attempts Towards the Molecular Analysis of Etiology and Pathogenesis of These Systemic Rheumatic Diseases

H.-J. Lakomek[1], and M. Schwochau[2]

[1]Medizinische Klinik und Poliklinik, Heinrich-Heine-Universität Düsseldorf,
4000 Düsseldorf 1, FRG
[2]Institut für Genetik, Heinrich-Heine-Universität Düsseldorf, 4000 Düsseldorf 1, FRG

Low concitivity of the commonly applied clinical criteria render the diagnosis of rheumatic diseases in general rather difficult, particularly in the early stages of these disorders. The identification of serological parameters specific for a particular disease would allow an earlier diagnosis with higher diagnostic confidence and open the way for a molecular analysis of the underlying pathomechanisms.

Investigating a set of xenotypic and homotypic antigen pools by immunoblotting techniques we were able to identify autoantibodies specific for AS and RA respectively.

Total protein preparations of insect tissues (Kc_0 cells of Drosophila melanogaster) contain at least four different antigens (36, 45, 52, and 74 k) reacting with antibodies present in sera of AS patients. The sera of these patients contain additional antibodies reacting specifically with the 93 D heat shock puff of D. *mel.* polytene chromosome preparations. Employing cytoimmunofluorescence and immunoblotting techniques AS associated antibodies were found in 82% of all AS patients and patients with suspected AS.

Concentrating on the most prominent reaction we further characterized and purified the 36 k antigen in order to isolate the respective antibody, which in turn is used to identify the corresponding human antigens.

Total protein preparations of human tissues (synovia, lymphocytes, and HeLa S3 cells) contain a 68 k antigen reacting with antibodies present in the sera of 64% (n = 84) of RA patients (diagnosed according to the ARA criterial). None of the sera of apparently healthy (n = 55) and only 6% of the sera of other arthrophaties (n = 82) (AS, reactive arthritis, SLE, PSS, overlap SLE/PSS, morphea, and OA) contained this antibody.

The 68 k antigen detected by the RA specific antibodies was further characterized (IEP: 5.1), purified and isolated, rendering the application of an ELISA technique for a specific and quantitative estimation of this antibody feasable.

The antibody against the 68 k antigen can readily be eluted from immunoblots thus opening the way to immunoscreening of the gene coding for the 68 k antigen from an appropriate cDNA expression library.

Characterization of the snRNP Protein N: Description of a Potential Sm Epitope

M. R. Lerner, G. McAllister, C. Schmauss, S. G. Amara, and A. Roby-Shemkovitz

Yale University, Section of Medical Neurobiology, School of Medicine, 333 Cedar Street, New Haven, CT 06510, USA

N is a highly conserved, Sm-epitope bearing, snRNP-associated protein found predominantly in brain. The amino acid sequences of N from humans and rats are identical. N is closely related to, but distinct from, the major Sm epitope bearing snRNP protein B (work of J. HARDIN et al.). In particular, N lacks a continuous sequence of 50 amino acids present near the carboxy terminus of B. Although the snRNP proteins B and B′ are generally expressed in all human cells, only N and B, but not B′ are present in human brain. Polyclonal antibodies raised against a 23 amino acid synthetic peptide based on part of the sequence of N recognize A, N, B and B′ on immunoblots. These antibodies can be used to immunoprecipitate the Sm class of U snRNAs from cell extracts.

Antigenic Structure of U snRNPS and Experimental Induction of Anti-U snRNP Autoantibodies in Mice

R. Lührmann

Institut für Molekularbiologie und Tumorforschung der Philipps-Universität, Emil-Mannkopff-Straße 2, D-3550 Marburg, FRG

Systemic lupus erythematosus (SLE) and related connective tissue diseases are generalized autoimmune diseases characterized by the production of autoantibodies against a variety of nuclear components. Among these are the anti-Sm and anti-RNP antibodies, which react with the protein moiety of the small nuclear RNPs containing the snRNAs U1, U2, U4, U5 and U6. Protein analyses of the snRNPs led to the identification, besides the seven proteins B′, B, D, D′, E, F and G common to these particles, of several particle-specific polypeptides. Thus, U1 RNP possesses in addition the proteins 70 K, A and C: U2 contains the proteins A′ and B″, and U5 contains a number of unique proteins characterised by apparent mol. wts. of 40, 52, 100, 102, 116 and 200 kDa. The latter particle, is the biggest snRNP and sediments at 20 S.

The antigenic determinants reacting with anti-RNP autoantibodies are located on the U 1 RNP-specific proteins 70 K, A and C, while the major immunoreactive Sm proteins are B', B and D. Antibodies against the common proteins E, F and G, as well as against the other snRNP-specific proteins including some of the U 5 specific proteins, also occur in some patient sera, but they are much less abundant.

The morphology of purified U 1 RNPs and the distribution of the RNP- and Sm-antigenic proteins at the surface of the U 1 RNP particle has been examined in the electron microscope by negative staining. U 1 RNP exhibits distinctive structural features, i.e. two characteristic protuberances 4 − 7 nm long and 3 − 4 nm wide that emerge from a central body about 8 nm in diameter. Electron microscopy of individual U 1 RNP particles gradually depleted of their specific proteins revealed, that the RNP antigenic proteins 70 K and A are contained in the two U 1 protuberances, while the round shaped body of the particel represents the core RNP structure encompassing the Sm proteins. Similar studies have been performed with the 20 S U 5 RNP particles which shows an overall elongated shape, about 23 nm long and 10 nm wide.

The antigenic structure of U 1 snRNP has further been studied by immunizing genetically nonautoimmune mice with isolated U 1 RNP particles. The antibody pattern produced by the mice was found to resemble the anti-RNP and anti-Sm autoimmune response in SLE patients closely. Not only were the major RNP- and Sm-antigenic proteins also predominantly immunogenic in the mice but they produced antibodies against the same regions on the antigenic polypeptides as do patients during the autoimmune response. This was verified by competitive binding studies with monoclonal antibodes derived from the mice as well as by mapping the autoimmunizing B cell epitopes using recombinant DNA approaches. These data suggest that the human autoantibody response is driven by endogeneous UsnRNP particles.

Autoantibodies to nucleolar components are a common serological feature of patients suffering from scleroderma, a collagen vascular autoimmune disease. While animal models, which spontaneously develop abundant anti-nuclear antibodies, have not yet been described, high titers of such antibodies may be induced by treating susceptible strains of mice with mercuric chloride. In collaboration with the group of Dr. E. GLEICHMANN (Düsseldorf), the major nucleolar autoantigen against which the $HgCl_2$-induced IgG autoantibodies from mice of strain B 10.S are directed, has been identified. It is a protein of apparent molecular weight of 36 kDa and pI value of about 8.6 which is associated with the nucleolar snRNA U 3, and by these criteria, must be identical with a polypeptide called fibrillarin. It is striking that scleroderma patients spontaneously produce autoantibodies against the same U 3 RNP protein. Our results provide a basis to investigate at the molecular level whether similar immunoregulatory dysfunctions may lead to the preferential anti-U 3 RNP autoantibody production in the animal model and in scleroderma patients.

The U1 RNBA Binding Site of the U1 snRNP-Associated A Protein Overlaps an Anti-U1 RNA Antibody Binding Site

C. Lutz-Freyermuth and J. D. Keene

Department of Microbiology and Immunology, Duke University Medical Center, Durham, NC 27710, USA

The U snRNPs are small nuclear ribonucleoprotein complexes that are known to be involved in the processing of precursor mRNAs to the mature form. Each snRNP is composed of both proteins unique to that snRNP as well as proteins common to all snRNPs. Some autoimmune patients make antibodies against these proteins, providing useful reagents to study the snRNPs. The precise protein-RNA and protein-protein interactions that exist in each snRNP are largely unknown.

proposed model for origin of anti-U1 RNA antibodies

We have previously described a unique human anti-RNA autoantibody found in patients with lupus overlap syndrome and rheumatoid arthritis (DEUTSCHER and KEENE, 1988, PNAS USA 85:3299–3303). The recognition site of this antibody on U1 RNA may overlap a binding site for another U1 RNA-associated protein. We propose that the anti-U1 RNA autoantibody is anti-idiotypic to an antibody directed against an RNA-binding domain of a U1-associated protein. Thus, it is likely that the anti-U1 RNA antibody was formed against the original autoantibody rather than by direct presentation of the naked U1 RNA to the immune system. Lymphocytes from the patient with this unique reactivity were isolated, immortalized with EBV, and were screened for the production of anti-U1 RNA antibodies that were devoid of any other reactivity. Antibodies with specificity to the second stem-loop structure of U1 RNA have been produced in this manner in order to address the origin of the antibody as an anti-idiotype.

This anti-U1 RNA patient serum also contains antibodies that react with the U1 snRNP-associated A protein. The A protein may bind to U1 RNA at the same or a similar site as does the U1 RNA-specific antibody. If this is true, the A protein and the U1 RNA-specific antibody should overlap and compete with one another for binding to the RNA. To examine this question, we have shown that the A protein will bind to U1 RNA in the absence of any other protein. We report the binding of the 32 kD A protein to stem-loop II of U1 RNA (nucleotides 49–85) as determined by Northwestern blotting assays and soluble protein *in vitro* binding assays (LUTZ-FREYERMUTH and KEENE, Mol. Cell Biol., in press). This binding site of the A protein on U1 RNA is found in a region with similarity to U2 RNA. The region of similarity in U2 RNA exists in a region that has been proposed to interact with a U2-associated protein, B″ (MATTAJ and DE ROBERTIS, 1985, Cell **40**:111–118). Proteins A and B″ are very similar at the amino acid level (SILLEKENS et al., 1987, EMBO J. **12**:3841–3848), and each contains two repeats of a proposed RNA recognition motif (RRM) that are likely to be involved in RNA binding. These findings suggest that structural similarities shared by U1 and U2 snRNPs may be involved in RNA-protein interactions within the spliceosome. Thus, we have shown that the A protein and the anti-U1 RNA antibody share overlapping binding sites on U1 RNA. These findings may have important implications for anti-idiotypic models of autoimmunity.

Anti-Ribosomal P Protein Antigens and Antibodies

J. Magsaam[1], H. Weissbach[2], N. Brot[2], and K. B. Elkon[1]

[1] The Hospital for Special Surgery, Cornell Medical Center 535 East 70th Street, New York, NY 10021, USA

[2] Roche Institute of Molecular Biology, Roche Research Center, Nutley, NJ 07110, USA

Approximately 12% of patients with SLE have anti-P and the presence of this antibody is relatively specific for the disease. A similar percentage (10%) of MRL/lpr mice, but not BXSB or NZB/W mice, also have anti-P antibodies. In humans with SLE, the presence of anti-P is strongly associated with a clinical subset of neuropsychiatric lupus.

The fine specificity of anti-P antibodies has been mapped by partial proteolysis, synthetic peptides and deletion mutants of a cDNA encoding the P2 protein. The results of these studies indicate that (i) there are linear and conformational epitope(s), (ii) there is a single linear epitope located within the C-terminal

22 amino acids present on all 3 P proteins, (iii) all sera recognize the C-terminal 11 residues but there is heterogeneity in binding to the C-terminal 7 residues, (iv) humans sera show similar binding to synthetic peptides composed of the human or A. salina amino acid sequences, (v) the C-terminal 22 amino acids are also the immunodominant epitope recognized by MRL/lpr sera.

To determine, whether the epitope recognized by anti-P is functionally important, F(ab')$_2$ or IgG containing anti-P activity was added to rabbit reticulocytes programmed with globin mRNA *in vitro* or was microinjected into the cytoplasm of WI 38 cells in culture. In both systems, anti-P, but not control IgG preparations, completely abolished protein synthesis. It seems probable therefore that the immunodominant epitope recognized by anti-P plays a critical role in factor-ribosome interaction.

Finally, to determine what role the antigens play in anti-P production, we compared the predicted amino acid sequences of the autoantigen in peripheral blood mononuclear cells from patients with anti-P and normal controls. cDNA was specifically primed with an oligonucleotide complimentary to the 3'-region of P 2, subcloned into lambda gt 11 and sequenced. No differences in the nucleotide sequences of the cDNA encoding the P 2 antigen were observed in the two groups. Although this observation makes a primary sequence abnormality unlikely, it does not exclude a role for the antigen in autoantibody induction or perpetuation.

Molecular Identification of the M 2 Antigens of Primary Biliary Cirrhosis

I. R. Mackay[1], M. E. Gershwin[2], M. J. Rowley[1], R. Uibo[1], and C. C. A. Bernard[3]

[1]Centre for Molecular Biology and Medicine, Monash University, Clayton, Victoria, 3168, Australia
[2]Department of Medicine, University of California at Davis, CA, USA
[3]Brain-Behaviour Research Institute, La Trobe University, Bundoora, Victoria, 3982, Australia

In 1957 the application of a complement fixation test using human tissues led to primary biliary cirrhosis (PBC) being recognized as an autoimmune disease. In 1965 this reactivity was specified by immunofluorescence as anti-mitochondrial, and subsequently the reactant was localized to the inner mitochondrial membrane. In 1985 immunoblotting showed that the mitochondrial (M 2) antigen was represented by two major polypeptides, 70–74 kDa and 45–52 kDa. In 1987 the molecular cloning of a cDNA sequence for an M2 antigen was reported, by antibody screening of a cDNA expression library (λgt 11). The cloned DNA (1370 bp) coded for a polypeptide which expressed the antigenic reactivity of the 70–74 kDa antigen. The amino acid sequence of the 70–74 kDa polypeptide was found to correspond with that of the E2 subunit of the mitochondrial pyruvate dehydrogenase (PDH) enzyme complex. PDH is a member of a family of three enzymes, the 2-oxo-acid dehydrogenases; the others are branched-chain, 2-oxo-acid dehydrogenase and 2-oxo-glutaric dehydrogenase and these contribute to the 45–52 kDa antigenic reactivity on Western blotting with PBC sera. These enzymes are abundant in nature and there are provocative sequence homologies in yeast and bacteria.

Deductions based on sequence conservation, and studies by absorption of antibody activity by synthetic peptides, placed an autoepitope (major immunogenic region) of PHD-E2 at residues 83–92, these being ile-glu-thr-asp-lys-ala-thr-ile-gly-phe-(IETDKATIGF). The lysine is the point of attachment of a prosthetic group, lipoic acid, essential for the function. The immunochemical reactions of PBC sera have a functional correlate in that diluted sera (1/50) will very rapidly, and with high specificity, inhibit the catalytic activity of the PDH enzyme on the natural substrate pyruvate, using a spectrophotometric readout of the formation of NADH. Rabbits immunized with the recombinant M2 protein, and Lewis rats immunized with a synthetic peptide corresponding to the autoepitope IET-DKATIGF, produced mitochondrial antibodies, but these sera did not inhibit PDH enzyme activity.

Thus there is evidence for a conformational or site difference in the epitope for natural and experimentally induced antibodies to the M2 mitochondrial (PDH-E2) autoantigen of PBC.

Molecular Biological Identification of Autoantigens in Autoimmune Hepatitis – Relevance for Pathogenesis, Diagnosis, and Treatment

M. P. Manns

Dept. of Medicine I, University of Mainz, Mainz, FRG

Several autoantigens are recognized by circulating autoantibodies in autoimmune liver diseases. Screening of cDNA libraries with human autoantibodies led to the molecular cloning of mitochondrial autoantigens in primary biliary cirrhosis (PBC) [1] and a microsomal antigen (LKM-1) in autoimmune hepatitis [2]. Antimitochondrial antibodies (AMA) in PBC react with subunits of the pyruvate dehydrogenase complex while LKM1 antibodies react with human cytochrome P450 db1. LKM-1 autoantibodies characterize a subgroup of autoimmune type chronic active hepatitis which can be distinguished serologically from classical autoimmune type "lupoid" hepatitis associated with antinuclear antibodies (ANA) and a third subgroup associated with antibodies to a soluble liver antigen (SLA) [3]. LKM-1 autoantibodies affinity purified from LKM-1-cDNA derived fusion protein recognize a 50 kD protein of liver as well as kidney microsomes. LKM-1 antibodies against P450 db1 are almost exclusively of subclass IgG1. A sensitive and specific diagnostic test based on LKM-1-cDNA derived fusion protein was developed for differential diagnosis of chronic hepatitis, namely to distinguish LKM-1 associated autoimmune hepatitis from virus induced liver diseases. In contrast to virus induced liver diseases autoimmune hepatitis profits from immunosuppression. LKM-1 specifically inhibit the function of P450 db1 *in vitro* [4]. P450 db1 is known to metabolize several drugs, such as debrisoquin, bufuralol and sparteine. Due to a genetic polymorphism, 10% of the normal caucasian population are deficient for this protein and are phenotypically slow metabolizers. Patients with LKM1 antibody positive liver disease express db1 protein in their liver, their sera inhibit the enzyme function *in vitro* but not P450 db1 catalysed drug metabolism *in vivo*. Thus autoantibodies reacting with the active site of an enzyme inhibit its function *in vitro* without affecting its drug metabolism *in vivo*. Possibly these findings serve as a model for other autoimmune disorders. The availability of specific cDNA's allows now a precise identification of the autoepitopes and facilitates new possibilities to study T-cell response.

References

1. GERSHWIN, N. E., MACKAY, I. R., STURGESS, A. et al. (1987): Identification and specificity of a cDNA encoding the 70 kD mitochondrial antigen recognized in primary biliary cirrhosis. J. Immunol. **138**, 3525
2. MANNS, M., JOHNSON, E. F., GRIFFIN, I. C. J., TAN, E. M., SULLIVAN, K. F. (1989): The major target of liver kidney microsomal autoantibodies in idiopathic autoimmune hepatitis is cytochrome P450 db1. J. Clin. Invest. **83**, 1066–1972
3. MANNS, M., GERKEN, G., KYRIATSOULIS, A., STARITZ, M., MEYER ZUM BÜSCHENFELDE, K.-H. (1987): Characterisation of a new subgroup of autoimmune chronic active hepatitis by autoantibodies against a soluble liver antigen. Lancet **1**, 292–294
4. ZANGER, U. M., HAURI, H. P., LOEPER, J., HOMBERG, J.-C., MEYER, U. A. (1988): Antibodies against human cytochrome P450 db1 in autoimmune hepatitis type II. Proc. Natl. Acad. Sci. USA, **27**, 8256–8260

Aminoacyl-tRNA Synthetases: an Overview

M. B. Mathews

Cold Spring Harbor Laboratory, P.O. Box 100, Cold Spring Harbor, New York, N.Y. 11724, USA

Antibodies directed against tRNA-related antigens are common in the inflammatory muscle diseases, polymyositis and dermatomyositis, but are relatively rare in other autoimmune diseases such as lupus and rheumatoid arthritis. Myositis patients also possess antibodies directed against nuclear antigens, such as RNP. The overall frequency of autoantibodies in myositis patients is approximately 90%. About a third of myositis patients carry antibodies against tRNA-related antigens, and this frequency is doubled in patients who also suffer from interstitial lung disease. Other kinds of autoantibodies, directed against DNA binding (Ku) and unidentified (Mi-2 and PM-Scl) proteins, are also characteristic of myositis sera. To a limited extent, these antibodies seem to be characteristic of subsets of patients, although the clinical basis for this specificity remains obscure.

Most of the tRNA-related antigens are aminoacyl-tRNA synthetases. These enzymes catalyze the charging of tRNA with its cognate aminoacid. There are twenty such enzymes, each specific for an individual aminoacid and able to recognize all of the tRNAs that accept this aminoacid. During the course of the reaction a molecule of ATP is hydrolyzed to AMP and pyrophosphate. In myositis, about 25% of patients contain antibodies of the Jo-1 class, specific for histidyl-tRNA synthetase. Jo-1 antibody immunoprecipitates the synthetase enzmye together with associated $tRNA^{His}$ but no antibodies have been detected that are specific for the tRNA itself. The antibodies inhibit aminoacylation of tRNA with histidine, and accordingly block protein synthesis in a rabbit reticulocyte cell-free system. Antibodies directed against other synthetases are considerably rarer. PL-7 antibody reacts with threonyl-tRNA synthetase and is present in approximately 6% of myositis patients. Like Jo-1, PL-7 antibody is directed against the enzyme and coprecipitates the cognate tRNA. Interestingly, an experimental antibody raised against the same enzyme fails to coprecipitate $tRNA^{Thr}$, suggesting that the rabbit antibody either reacts with a denatured form of the protein incapable of binding tRNA or, alternatively, blocks tRNA binding to the enzyme. A third specificity, known as PL-12, precipitates both alanyl-tRNA and $tRNA^{Ala}$ but differs from the two previous specificities in two ways. The synthetase and the tRNA are recognized separately by autoantibodies directed against the protein and RNA components, and antibodies against the synthetase fail to coprecipitate the tRNA. The site on the tRNA that is recognized by the anti-$tRNA^{Ala}$ component has been identified as the anticodon stem and loop structure. PL-12 antibody is also found in about 5% of myositis patients. Additional specificities that have been detected are antibodies against isoleucyl- and glycyl-tRNA-synthetases, and antibodies against a moiety that is believed to be the protein synthesis elongation factor-1 (EF-1). Interestingly, patient's sera often contain more than one tpye of antibody, but no serum has yet been reported in which low or more of the tRNA related specificities coexist.

A New Autoantibody Specific for the Limited Systemic Sclerosis (lSSc) Found Through Molecular Biology

G. G. Maul, P. McGregory, D. Ziemnicka-Kotula, and C. Ascoli

The Wistar Institute of Anatomy and Biology, 36th Street at Spruce, Philadelphia, PA 19104, USA

Presently there are two relatively specific autoantibody systems recognized for systemic sclerosis (SSc). About 35% of patient sera with diffuse SSc recognize topoisomerase I and about 65% of lSSc recognize one or more of the three low-abundance proteins of the kinetochore. Proteins that are rare and present in structures similarly appearing in immunofluorescence will not be recognized by double immunodiffusion or immunoblotting. They may, however, be found through cloning.

During our attempts to clone the 140 kDa protein of the kinetochore we selected a clone recognized by several sera from lSSc patients. To determine the antigenic localization of the protein cloned we produced monoclonal antibodies against the fusion protein. The monoclonal antibody did not recognize the kinetochore. Instead it labeled new nuclear domain consisting of 8−16 variously sized precisely circumscribed dots. Double labeling proved that the antigen localization was not on the prekinetochore nor was it on the primary constriciton of chromosomes. The protein is translated from a 100 kDa in RNA and partial sequencing shows that it does not correspond to any known protein.

Immunohistochemical ultrastructural analysis lends credence to the observation that some of these dots appear as rings or hollow spheres, are present as pairs and may double during the cell cycle. Together with observations from other sera recognizing the same structure we conclude that we have cloned the first protein of a new nuclear domain for which a function has yet to be found.

Large scale screening showed that the new antibodies are lSSc-specific (65% of patients), that the kinetochore antibodies of SLE patients do not react with this antigen, that the sera of primary biliary cirrhosis patients are negative unless they have kinetochore autoantibodies (3/25) and specifically that the serum antibodies of dSSc patients do not react with this antigen (0/55). In 100 sera from Red cross volunteers we found one serum positive for these specific dots by immunofluorescence but it was negative with the cloned antigen. The minor overlap recognized with PBC patients sera corresponds to the kinetochore and may select patients with an overlap syndrome.

Determination of an Epitope of the Diffuse Scleroderma Marker Antigen Topoisomerase I. Sequence Similarity with Retroviral p30^{gag} Protein Suggests a Possible Cause for Autoimmunity in Scleroderma

G. G. Maul, S. A. Juminez, and D. Ziemnicka-Kotula

Wistar Institute of Anatomy and Biology, 36th and Spruce Streets, Philadelphia, PA 19104, USA
Department of Medicine Thomas Jefferson University, 1020 Locust Street, Philadelphia, PA 19107, USA

The possibility that viruses play a role in the etiology of various autoimmune diseases has been proposed. One approach to the search for these agents involves identifying potential crossreactive epitopes in viruses that infect cells of the immune system or of the target tissues. Anti-topoisomerase I antibodies are the marker autoantibodies for diffuse systemic sclerosis (dSSc). The major epitope of the antigen was therefore sought through cloning and sequencing of the cDNA for human topoisomerase I and eventually by the synthesis of the smallest possible peptide recognized by sera from patients with the diffuse form of systemic sclerosis. Of two potential antigenic 11 amino acid sequences one contained 6 sequential amino acids that are identical to a sequence present in the group-specific antigen (p30^{gag}) of some mammalian retroviruses. This sequence was recognized by many dSSc patients sera. It is separated by only one amino acid from the retroviral epitope sequence that crossreacts with autoantibodies against the mixed connective-tissue disease and systemic lupus erythromatosus marker antigen (U$_1$) RNP (60 kDa). These findings suggest that a retroviral agent may be involved in the pathogenesis of scleroderma, and other connective tissue diseases and that antibodies to intracellular autoantigens are not involved in the pathogenesis of autoimmune disease but may be useful as footprints for tracking the potential etiological agent of autoimmune disease.

The Spectrum of Antinuclear Antibodies (ANA) and Clinical Findings in Children with Anti-U 1-RNP Antibodies

H. Michels[1], H. O. Kettner[1], H. Truckenbrodt[1], and E. Genth[2]

[1]Rheumatic Children's Hospital, Garmisch-Partenkirchen, FRG
[2]Rheumatic Research Institute, Rheumatic Hospital, Aachen, FRG

Since 1977 we have had 30 patients (23 ♀, 7 ♂) with anti-U 1-RNP antibodies. All had high titer ANA with a speckled pattern. 19 of the 30 patients had only anti-U 1-RNP antibodies, 11/30 were found with antibodies to further nuclear antigens:

3 patients to dsDNA,
1 patient to dsDNA and Sm
1 patient to dsDNA, Sm and to S cl-70
3 patients to Sm
1 patient to Sm and SS-A
1 patient to Sm, SS-A and SS-B
1 patient to SS-A

Mean age at onset of disease was 8.4 years, 19/30 had Raynaud's phenomenon, 13/30 recurrent parotid gland enlargements. 24/30 showed skin alterations, often unspecific maculopapulous exanthema, possible skleroderma-like skin alterations during further course (13/30). Indication for admission was usually arthritis/arthralgia, mostly from beginning (48%) as polyarthritis.
The arthritis can be deforming, rarely erosive (1/30).
Because of the frequent positive IgM-rheumatoid factor (RF) (21/30), accompanied in 7/21 by "rheumatic nodules", the RF-positive juvenile rheumatoid arthritis must be excluded.
Muscular weakness/myalgia were observed in 39%.
Notable laboratory findings are increased IgG levels (26/30 > 200 mg%, maximal 9440 mg%), often together with elevated total protein (14/26, maximal 12.4%) and also connected with raised plasma viscosity .

Prognosis depends upon the possible organ manifestations (kidney, lung, central nervous system, heart), seems to be favourable, however, quoad vitam in most cases. So far we have had two fatal cases, a 14-year old girl with "acute heart failure" after 8 years disease duration and one 24 year old patient (low titer anti-U 1-RNP and high titer anti-dsDNA) who died at the age of 25 years, 15 years after onset of disease during renal transplantation rejection (condition after renal insufficiency through membranoproliferative glomerulonephritis).

It seems that the titer level of anti-U 1-RNP antibodies and the spectrum of ANA bear significance for the extent of the clinical symptomatology.

Molecular Cloning of the Human Autoantigen KU (p70/p80), a DNA-Terminal-Binding Protein Complex

T. Mimori[1], N. Hama[1], A. Suwa[1], Y. Ohsone[1], M. Akizuki[1], M. Homma[1], A. J. Griffith[2], and J. A. Hardin[2]

[1] Keio University School of Medicine, Tokyo, Japan
[2] Yale University School of Medicine, New Haven, Connecticut, USA

Anti-Ku autoantibodies in patients with PSS-PM overlap syndrome recognize a 70 kD/80 kD protein heterodimer which binds selectively to terminal region of dsDNA. In the present study, we isolated and characterized cDNA clones that encode the Ku autoantigen, and intended to use them for clinical application.

In the first step, a human hepatoma cell cDNA library inserted into the EcoRI site of $\lambda gt11$ phages were screened with an anti-Ku serum to identify plaques expressing Ku epitopes. Three positive clones (K14, K68 and K71) were isolated and demonstrated to express fusion proteins recognized by anti-Ku antibodies. In the second step, OKAYAMA-BERG cDNA library was screened by using an isolated cDNA encoding the partial 80kD-Ku sequence (K71) as a probe for colony hybridization. The clone Ku80-6 that contained the longest cDNA insert (3.4 kb, identical with the larger mRNA from two mRNAs hybridized by K71) was isolated, and its nucleotide sequence was determined by SANGER's dideoxy method. The Ku80-6 cDNA contained a single long open reading frame encoding 732 amino acids (Mr = 82713) followed by 1081 bases of 3'-non-coding region and a poly(A) tail. The putative polypeptide contained a Leu-Ser repeat in every 7 amino acid residue which may contribute the formation of "Leucine zipper". The sequence of the Ku80-6 was compared with previously described sequences using the computer search, but no significant homology was found either in DNA (GenBank) or protein (NBRF) data bank. In Southern blot, the Ku80-6 hybridized with 4–5 DNA bands from human leukocyte DNA digested with various restriction enzymes. It was noted that RFLP was seen in the 2.8 kb-HindIII fragment and likely to associate with SLE patients who had anti-U1-RNP antibodies. Using purified fusionproteins expressing from K14 (70 kD) and K71 (80 kD) clones, we developed ELISA to detect anti-Ku antibodies. When sera from various collagen diseases were screened by this assay, anti-Ku antibodies were mostly detected in patients with overlap syndrome, consistent with the result of a conventional immunodiffusion assay.

Our cDNA encoding the Ku antigenic proteins will be a powerful tool to study not only the structure and function of the Ku autoantigen but also pathogenetic mechanisms of autoimmune diseases.

Autoantibodies to a Histone Cross-Reactive DNA-Binding Protein of M$_r$ 110000 in Systemic Lupus Erythematosus and Other Diseases and in Autoimmune Mice

S. Minota, W. N. Jarjour, R. A. S. Roubey, T. Mimura, and J. B. Winfield

Division of Rheumatology and Immunology, University of North Carolina at Chapel Hill, Chapel Hill, NC 27514, USA

This investigation characterizes a novel 110 kD autoantigen (110 K) recognized by autoantibodies in serum from patients with systemic lupus erythematosus (SLE) or certain other autoimmune or viral diseases, and MRL/Mp-lpr/lpr mice. IgM and, less frequently, IgG autoantibodies to this protein were detected by one- and two-dimensional immunoblotting and by immunoprecipitation utilizing non-ionic detergent lysates of various human lymphoid and non-lymphoid cells. By immunoblotting, 110 K was shown to be an intracellular DNA-binding protein of pI 5.4, containing at least one phosphotyrosyl residue. In cell fractionation experiments, 110 K was present in both the nucleus and the cytosol, but not in plasma membranes or mitochondria. PHA stimulation appeared to increase the amount of 110 K in peripheral T lymphocytes, suggesting that cellular activation either increased the expression of the antigen or altered its structure such that antibody reactivity was enhanced. Certain SLE sera with pre-formed DNA/anti-DNA complexes also reacted with 110 K in immunoblots via DNA-110 K binding. Autoantibodies to 110 K were distinguished from DNA/anti-DNA complexes by retention of 110 K-binding activity in sera subjected to DNase I digestion and in IgM purified by sucrose density gradient ultracentrifugation under immune complex disassociating conditions. IgM anti-110 K antibodies in SLE sera were associated in all but two instances with antibodies to histone H1. Linkage of anti-110 K with antibodies to histone H2B was demonstrated as well. Affinity purification of anti-110 K and anti-histone antibodies revealed that this relationship was due, in part, to antibody cross-reactivity. Considerable evidence was obtained to suggest that 110 K was distinct from hsp 110, a stress protein, and from already-defined autoantigens of approximately the same size, i.e., topoisomerase I, PM-Scl, and RNA polymerase I.

IgM autoantibodies to 110 K were particularly prevalent in childhood SLE (15/15, 100%), acute hepatitis A infection (16/20, 80%), Sjögren's syndrome (17/24, 71%), adult SLE (27/42, 67%), and systemic sclerosis (7/16, 44%). Anti-110 K was detected less frequently in patients with infectious mononucleosis (4/20, 20%) or other rheumatic diseases: polymyositis (2/10, 20%), rheumatoid arthritis (1/20, 5%), polymyalgia rheumatica (1/20, 5%), and spondyloarthropathy (0/20). Anti-110 K antibodies were not demonstrable in serum from 10 normal individuals. In conclusion, the data suggest a special association of autoantibodies to a novel 110 kD nuclear/cytoplasmic protein with systemic autoimmune disease and certain viral infections.

cDNA Cloning and Expression of U1snRNP C Protein

Y. Misaki[1], K. Yamamoto[1], H. Miura[1], H. Fujii[1], K. Nishioka[2], and T. Miyamoto[1]

[1] Department of Medicine and Physical Therapy, Faculty of Medicine, University of Tokyo, Japan
[2] Institute of Rheumatology, Tokyo Women's Medical College, Tokyo, Japan

As previously reported, we have cloned a cDNA termed PS2 which encodes U1snRNP C protein (J. Immunol. 1988). Here we report the cloning and expression of a putative full lenght cDNA encoding the entire coding region of the U1snRNP C protein.

Using PS2 as a probe, we have screened cDNA libraries constructed from human fibroblasts by the Okayama-Berg method, which were found to contain many full-length cDNAs. After screening two different cDNA libraries, the longest cDNA insert hybridized with PS2 was 800 bp. We call this cDNA as FS2. In the Northern blotting using RNA from human PBC, nearly the same length of the band was identified. Sequencing of FS2 revealed that it contained the initiation codon in the long open reading frame. These results suggest that FS2 is a full-length cDNA encoding the U1snRNP C protein, although FS2 could encode only 15 kDa protein.

In order to express this cDNA in *E. coli*, we subcloned the insert into an expression vector, pEX. This vector produces a fusion protein with cro-β-galactosidase. Transformed *E. coli* was screened with anti-RNP positive sera. A single colony, FS2EX was identified to produce the fusion protein which was positive with the patients' sera. We are now trying to discriminate the epitope recognized by anti-RNP antibodies by generating the deletion mutants of this FS2EX.

Further Characterization of the Anti-Wa Antibody to a tRNA-Related Protein in Progressive Systemic Sclerosis

K. Miyachi[1], T. Mimori[2], S. Takano[1], H. Yamagata[3], Y. Matsuoka[4], S. Irimajiri[4], K. Tani[5], M. Akizuki[2], and M. Homma[2]

[1]Autoimmune Disease Center, Health Sciences Research Institute, Yokohama, Japan
[2]Department of Internal Medicine, Keio University, School of Medicine, Tokyo, Japan
[3]Department of Internal Medicine, National Eastern Murayama Hospital, Tokyo, Japan
[4]Department of Internal Medicine, Kawasaki Municipal Hospital, Kawasaki, Japan
[5]Department of Internal Medicine, Yokohama City University Hospital, Yokohama, Japan

In 1985, YAMAGATA reported on a new antibody (anti-Wa Ab) to one of the tRNA related proteins in a patient with progressive systemic sclerosis (PSS). Since then however further studies concerning this antibody have not been reported. This present study identifies four other PSS patients with serum anti-Wa Ab. This antibody was detected by double immunodiffusion using calf thymus extract and human liver supernatant, but not by indirect immunofluorescence with mouse kidney section of HEp II cells. When immunoblotting was conducted on the antigen preparation following SDS-PAGE and electrophoretic transfer to nitrocellulose membrane, a band appeared at the 45 kd position. In addition, the four sera were found to precipitate ^{32}P-labelled HeLa cell tRNA but not UsnRNA.

Clinical manifestations of 4 PSS patients with anti-Wa antibody

Hospital	Kawasaki Municipal Hospital		Yokohama City University Hospital	
Patient	KT	MF	MM	YT
Age	49	64	64	47
Sex	f	f	f	f
Duration of Raynaud' ph. (v)	7	19	3	2
Skin	sclero.	acro.	acro.	sclero.
Lung	–	fibrosis	lung cancer	–
Heart	–	cardiomegaly	–	cardiomegaly
Gastrointestinal	–	intestinal dilatation	esophageal hernia	–
Articular	finger joint pain	–	–	–
Myalgia	+	–	–	–

sclero, sclerodactylia; *acro*, acrosclerosis

The anti-Wa Ab was observed in 3% (4/130) of patients with PSS, but not in 600 patients with systemic lupus erythematosus. This antibody was not associated with other marker antibodies seen in PSS such as anti-Scl 70 and anti-centromere antibodies. None of the four PSS patients had myositis except one patient who complained of mild myalgia. At present those patients do not show clinical overlap feature of PSS and polymyositis/dermatomyositis. Summary of clinical manifestation is as shown on page 56.

Characteristics and Interrelation of Autoantibodies in Scleroderma Sera

Y. Moroi

Dept. of Internal Medicine and Physical Therapy, University of Tokyo, Tokyo, Japan

Several kinds of autoantibodies against cellular components have been so far characterized and proved to be specific in various degree for the patient with scleroderma. These include antibodies against topoisomerase I (TopoI), centromere, nRNP, nucleolus, mitochondria, centriole and mitotic spindle.

We analyzed immunoglobulin class and titer of anti-TopoI by ELISA using chemically purified TopoI as antigen. Anti-centromere antibody was also analyzed by indirect immunofluorescence (IF) method.

All the scleroderma sera which contained anti-Scl 70 antibody by double-immunodifusion (DID) showed positive IgG anti-TopoI by ELISA. About 60% of these sera also contained IgA class antibody, but no IgM antibody was detected. Same tendency was observed in case of anti-centromere antibody, namely IgG anti-centromere in all the sera, IgA antibody in about 60% and IgM antibody in less than 30% of the sera which was positive anti-centromere by FITC-anti globulin. Interrelation of these antibodies including anti-centromere, centriole and mitotic spindle will be discussed.

Characterisation of an Autoantigen in Graves' Hyperthyroidism

A. F. Mulcahy and A. G. Diamond

Medical Molecular Biology Group, Medical School, University of Newcastle-Upon-Tyne, Framlington Place, Newcastle-Upon-Tyne, NE2 4HH, UK

GRAVES' Hyperthyroidism is an autoimmune condition in which antibodies are produced against several thyroid components. At least three autoantigens have been described in human thyroid; thyroid stimulating hormone receptor (TSH-R), thyroglobulin (Tg) and thyroid peroxidase (TPO). Of these, only the Tg and TPO autoantigens have been well characterised.

To further identify autoantigens involved in GRAVES' Hyperthyroidism a cDNA library was constructed in the $\lambda gt11$ vector from thyroid polyA$^+$ RNA from a GRAVES' Hyperthyroidism patient who had not received anti-thyroid drugs prior to surgery. The cDNA library was screened with a serum from a different GRAVES' patient. One strongly positive clone, TM17.1, from this screening has been studied further. TM17.1 has been tested for reactivity with a limited number of sera and was found to be positive with other GRAVES' sera, but negative with two HASHIMOTO's sera and control sera. The clone contains a 3.7 kb cDNA insert with a single internal EcoR1 site producing fragments of 3 kb and 0.7 kb. Northern blot analysis of thyroid RNA showed that both fragments identify RNA approximately 3.7 kb in length, consistent with the clone containing a single cDNA species of, or near, full length. This RNA was not present in B lymphoblastoid cell lines. Southern blot analysis of human genomic DNA using the 3 kb and 0.7 kb EcoR1 fragments produced few bands, implying that the clone was a product of a single gene or a low copy number family. The 0.7 kb fragment has been sequenced and shows no significant homology with entries in the Genbank database (Release 55). Therefore, TM17.1 is neither of the known thyroid-specific antigens (Tg, TPO). It shows no homology with the recently described 70 kDa autoantigen with TSH-binding properties (CHAN et al., J. Biol. Chem. **264**:3651, 1989) nor a second autoantigen encoding a protein related to the mitochondrial solute carrier protein (L. D. KOHN; personal communication).

Further work is in progress on the extent of antibody reactivity in patient groups and the tissue distribution of the antigen, the complete sequence determination and whether T-lymphocyte reactivity to the protein can be detected in this disease.

Clinical Significance of Anti-Ubiquitin Antibodies in Systemic Lupus Erythematosus

S. Muller, P. Joubaud, J. P. Briand, S. Plaué, and M. H. V. Van Regenmortel

Laboratoire d'Immunochimie, Institut de Biologie Moléculaire et Cellulaire, CNRS, Strasbourg, France

Antibodies to ubiquitin and to ubiquitinated histones have been found in the sera of patients with systemic lupus erythematosus (SLE) using an enzyme-linked immunosorbent assay (ELISA) and immunoblotting experiments [1]. In ELISA, the reaction could be measured with ubiquitin and with synthetic peptides corresponding either to residues 22–45 of the ubiquitin molecule or to the branched moiety of ubiquitinated histone H2A (T peptides).

The pathogenic and clinical significance of antibodies to ubiquitin in SLE remains unclear. In an attempt to correlate the presence of these autoantibodies with the clinical pattern of disease, the appearance of IgG antibodies reacting with whole ubiquitin and synthetic fragments was measured in SLE patients at different stages of the disease. The results were compared to those obtained by measuring the reactivity of sera to usual SLE markers such as native double-stranded DNA and Sm. Our findings indicate that the presence of antibodies to ubiquitin correlates with specific clinical phases of the disease and that they could represent an early marker for SLE.

Reference

1. MULLER, S., BRIAND, J. P., VAN REGENMORTEL, M. H. V. (1988): Presence of antibodies to ubiquitin during the autoimmune response associated with systemic lupus erythematosus. Proc. Natl. Acad. Sci. USA **85**, 8176–8180

The Natural History of PCNA/Cyclin

P. K. Nakane

Department of Anatomy, Nagasaki University School of Medicine, Nagasaki, Japan

PCNA/cyclin was originally described in proliferating mammalian cells as a nuclear protein with an apparent molecular weight of 33000–36000 and was recently found to be a DNA polymerase-delta auxiliary protein. When the cDNA for PCNA/cyclin was cloned and analyzed, both in the rat and human, it was found that the protein consisted of 261 amino acids with a calculated molecular weight of 28 700. The amino acid sequences of the rat and man PCNA/cyclin were the same, except the rat 7th amino acid Ile was Val in man; the 33rd, Gly was Ser; the 190th, Ser was Thr; and the 216th, Pro was Ser. The Southern blot analysis of rat and human genomic DNA indicated that there is one copy of PCNA/cyclin per haploid genome of the both species. The gene for PCNA/cyclin was assigned to a long arm of human chromosome 2 at 2q33. The rat PCNA/cyclin cDNA probe hybridized with homologous sequences in genomic DNAs from rice, soybean, tobacco and red pepper and when the PCNA/cyclin-related molecular clone isolated from rice DNA was used as a probe for RNA blot analysis, the probe hybridized with a 1.2 kilobase transcript in RNA from rice root tips and shoots. Immunohistochemically, in the proliferating cells, PCNA/cyclin first appeared in the cytoplasm, migrated into nuclei and again in the cytoplasm in the region of the Golgi complexes. With our study, at what exact stage of mitosis PCNA/cyclin re-entered cytoplasm could not be defined, we presume it was during the prophase since little or not PCNA/cyclin was associated with the metaphase chromosomes. The strong conservation of the gene and the protein for PCNA/cyclin among animal and plant kingdoms suggests the essential role of this protein in DNA replication in eukaryotes.

Identification of Several Independent Autoreactive Epitopes of the Human 68 kDa (U 1) snRNP-Autoantigen

H. J. Netter[1], H. H. Guldner[1], C. Szostecki[1], H. J. Lakomek[2], and H. Will[1]

[1]Max Planck Institut für Biochemie, 8033 Martinsried, FRG
[2]Medizinische Klinik C, 4000 Düsseldorf, FRG

We have recently isolated a human cDNA coding for the human (U 1) snRNP-specific 68 kDa autoantigen. Using the purified recombinant p 68 protein expressed in *E. coli* we established an ELISA-assay for p 68 autoantibody detection suitable for clinical routine [1]. Moreover, we recently identified three autoantigenic domains of the p 68 autoantigen [2].

To localize the autoreactive epitopes in more detail, to get an rough estimate on how many independent epitopes are recognized by anti-p68 autoantibodies, and whether patient specific patterns can be identified a detailed mapping of autoreactive determinants was performed with a collection of human autoimmune sera. Using a large series of fusion proteins in immunoblotting as well as peptide based ELISAs we identified several independent epitopes a few amino acids in length and larger sequences which presumably represent discontinuous epitopes. One of these epitopes is recognized by virtually all anti-p68 antibody positive sera, another one by appr. 30% and some reacted with less than 10% of the sera. Patient specific epitope recognition patterns were identified. These data demonstrate polyclonality of the anti-68 kDa autoimmune response, rule out somatic mutation as a sole mechanism of anti-68 kDa autoantibody induction, and argue for an antigen-driven autoimmune response but do not exclude the involvement of microorganisms as autoimmune process initiators by molecular mimicry. The identification of several independent autoreactive epitopes allows differential screening for patient specific epitope patterns which may become a useful tool for diagnosis, prognosis and therapy control.

References

1. NETTER, H. J., GULDNER, H. H., SZOSTECKI, C., LAKOMEK, H. J., WILL, H. (1988): A recombinant autoantigen derived from the human (U1) small nuclear RNP-specific 68-kd protein. Expression in Escherichia coli and serodiagnostic application. Arthritis Rheum. **31**, 616–621
2. GULDNER, H. H., NETTER, H. J., SZOSTECKI, C., LAKOMEK, H. J., WILL, H. (1988): Epitope mapping with a recombinant human 68-kDa (U1) ribonucleoprotein antigen reveals heterogeneous autoantibody profiles in human autoimmune sera. J. Immunol. **141**, 469–475

Current Ideas on Tolerance Mechanisms and Autoimmunity

G. J. V. Nossal

The Walter and Eliza Hall Institute of Medical Research, P. O. Royal Melbourne Hospital, Victoria 3050, Australia

The work of the last two years has seen some giant strides taken in our understanding of mechanisms of immunological tolerance. Extensive use of transgenic animals has provided new models of great power and elegance, though each model must be carefully analyzed for those features that might introduce artefacts. Through this work, it has become apparent that both positive selection for recognition of MHC and negative selection against high affinity anti-self reactivity (clonal abortion) go on within the thymus soon after CD4$^+$ CD8$^+$ T cells have displayed their T cell receptor molecules. Evidence is mounting that extrathymic mechanisms of T cell silencing (clonal anergy) can occur in the periphery if T cells encounter self antigens in the absence of help.

Tolerance to certain self antigens exists also within the B cell compartement. For important cell surface antigens, such as self MHC, clonal abortion within the bone marrow (analogous to thymic self-censorship) occurs. For soluble self antigens, clonal anergy may be induced in immature B cells. This effect has definite affinity thresholds, and some self antigens fail to induce measurable B cell tolerance.

Finally, some evidence exists that precursors of memory B cells go through a "second window" of tolerance susceptibility. Recent work from our laboratory suggests that in vivo administration of soluble antigen can abrogate the somatic V gene hypermutation in B cells that underlies affinity maturation. It seems likely that this mechanism breaks down in autoimmunity, as the pathogenic autoantibodies do display multiple mutations.

Molecular Cloning of a cDNA for the B Polypeptide of the U snRNPs

Y. Ohosone[1], T. Mimori[2], A. Griffith[1], M. Akizuki[2], M. Homma[2], J. Craft[1], and J. A. Hardin[1]

[1] Yale University, New Haven, CT 06510, USA
[2] Keio University, Tokyo, Japan

Anti-Sm antibodies are a dominant feature of the autoimmune response of SLE. These antibodies target epitopes found on the B'/B and D polypeptides of the U series snRNP particles. We have used sera containing this specificity to isolate and clone cDNA^{S3-4} (780 bases) which encodes approximately two thirds of polypeptide B.

To obtain a full length cDNA, we screened a human fibroblast cDNA library using cDNA^{S3-4} as a probe and isolated cDNA^B (1136 bases). Sequencing demonstrated a single open reading frame encoding a polypeptide of 285 amino acids, a size closely approximating the B polypeptide. The derived sequence is especially rich in proline residues and lacks the RNP consensus sequence and the RNA binding domain common to a number of RNA binding proteins − a finding consistent with the idea that the B polypeptides associate with U small RNAs indirectly through interaction with other polypeptides. Except for a 50 amino acid insert near its carboxy terminus, the cDNA^B sequence is nearly homologous at the aminoacid level with polypeptide N, a newly recognized tissue specific component of Sm snRNPs. Structural differences in B and N polypeptides may regulate tissue specific alternative splicing of mRNA. Several studies have been directed at understanding the relationship of the two B polypeptides. mRNAs which hybridize with cDNA^{S3-4} are translated in vitro into both polypeptides. In contrast, in vitro expression of the full length cDNA^B yields only the B polypeptide. These results suggest that there are two related, but independent mRNAs for B'/B.

Studies of individual autoantigenic epitopes demonstrate that anti-Sm antibodies eluted from the cDNA^{S3-4} fusion protein immunoprecipitate only the U 1 snRNP in some cases and all Sm snRNPs in others. This observation is consistent with the idea that cDNA^{S3-4} encodes two regions of the B polypeptide: one that is accessible to antibodies on the U 1 snRNP alone and another that is available for interaction on all of the Sm snRNPs.

The Induction of Anti-DNA Antibodies in Normal Mice by Immunization with Bacterial DNA

D. S. Pisetsky, J. P. Grudier, and G. S. Gilkeson

Division of Rheumatology and Immunology, Duke University Medical Center, Durham, NC 27705, USA

To investigate the role of DNA in the induction of anti-DNA antibodies in systemic lupus erythematosus (SLE), the immune response of mice to bacterial DNA was investigated. BALB/c mice immunized with E. coli (EC) single-stranded DNA (ssDNA) in complexes with mBSA produced antibody levels much greater than similar immunization with calf thymus (CT) DNA. The induced antibodies contained a population specific for EC DNA as well as a population crossreactive with CT as well as other DNAs. The induced antibodies bound moreover to a variety of synthetic polynucleotides including poly dC, poly I, and poly dI without reactivity to poly dT or poly dU. In contrast, immunization with double-stranded (ds) E. coli DNA elicited antibodies specific for ds E. coli DNA without crossreactivity to mammalian DNA.

Comparable results were obtained by immunization of mice with DNA from *Micrococcus lysodeikticus*. Together, these studies indicate that bacterial DNA contains regions that can be the target of antibody responses likely because they are rarely expressed in mammalian DNA. These regions could serve as a trigger for an anti-DNA response in SLE by a process of molecular mimicry.

The Binding of Anti-La Antibodies to Fusion Proteins Containing Various La Epitopes

D. S. Pisetsky, J. D. Keene, and E. W. St. Clair

Division of Rheumatology and Immunology, Duke University Medical Center, Durham, NC 27705, USA

To investigate the mechanisms underlying the anti-La autoantibody response, the fine specificity of anti-La antibodies was assessed using a series of recombinantly derived fusion proteins containing various portions of the La molecule. Using solid phase ELISAs, anti-La positive sera of patients with a variety of connective tissue diseases bound to fusion proteins representing the middle (LaC) as well as amino (LaA) and carboxyl (LaD) terminal portions of the La molecule. The quantitative binding to the different La fragments was independent of diagnosis and variable among patients with the same diagnosis. Affinity chromatography using solubilized fusion proteins attached to Sepharose indicated that antibodies binding to the different fragments were independent populations; thus, antibodies binding to a LaC column bound poorly to LaA or LaD by ELISA. Analysis of sequential sera of individuals indicated that antibody levels to the different fragments varied in parallel. Together, these observations suggest that anti-La antibodies recognize multiple epitopes on the La antigen and arise as an immune response to the La molecule itself.

Isolation and Sequencing of Human Lamin β cDNA: Mammalian Lamins A, B and C Contain Leucine Heptad Repeats

K. M. Pollard, E. Kl. Chan, B. J. Grant, K. F. Sullivan, E. M. Tan, and C. A. Glass

W M Keck Autoimmune Disease Center and DNA Coro Facility, Department of Molecular and Experimental Medicine and Department of Molecular Biology, Research Institute of Scripps Clinic, La Jolla, CA 92037, USA

The nuclear lamins A, B and C form a meshwork of filaments on the inner, or nucleoplasmic, surface of the nuclear envelope. Autoantibodies to all three mammalian lamins have been found in the serum of patients with certain immunological disorders such as systemic lupus erythematosus, scleroderma and autoimmune liver disease. These sera have proven useful reagents for the characterisation of lamins in mammalian and other species and for the cloning of human lamins A and C. In this report we describe our use of a NZB/W Fl mouse monoclonal autoantibody, called 72B9, to clone nuclear lamin B using a λgt11 cDNA expression library prepared from the human leukemia T cell line MOLT-4. A unique feature of this study is that the monoclonal antibody used reacts in immunofluorescence studies with the nucleolus and targets the 34 kDa protein component of the nucleolus restricted U3 small nuclear ribonucleoprotein particle (U3snRNP). The identity of the encoded protein as lamin B was established by both biochemical and immunological criteria which included immunoprecipitation of *in vitro* translated product of RNA transcripts of the cDNA by lamin B specific antibodies. Detection of mRNA in RL60 cells, that express only lamin B, or HeLa cells, that express all three major lamins A, B and C, and the colocalisation of *in vitro* translated product with HeLa cell lamin B by two-dimensional gel electrophoresis, strongly suggests that a single lamin B is expressed in mammalian somatic cells. Southern blot analysis revealed that a single gene encodes human lamin B. Inspection of the deduced amino acid sequence of lamin B revealed the presence in coil 1B of the α-helical domain of a leucine heptad repeat region. Leucine heptad repeats were also found in coil 1B of other lamins, including the type A lamins which also contain a leucine heptad repeat in coil 2 of the α-helical domain. These leucine heptad repeats are centrally located on coils 1B and 2, which suggests a role in the dimerisation of lamin monomers. The lamins therefore belong to the growing list of nuclear proteins whose dimerisation domains contain leucine heptad repeats.

Detection of Autoantibodies Using Recombinant Antigens

I. Pettersson, U. Nyman, E. Welin, and N. Ringertz

Department of Medical Cell Genetics, Karolinska Institutet, Stockholm, Sweden

The presence of high serum titers of anti-RNP antibodies, is a disease criterium for the autoimmune disease Mixed Connective Tissue Disease (MCTD), Anti-RNP antibodies are also detected in sera from patients with systemic lupus erythematosus (SLE), but usually with lower titers and in conjunction with another specificity, anti-Sm. Both types of antibodies react with intranuclear RNA-protein complexes involved in splicing, called the U snRNPs. Several studies have shown that anti-RNP antibodies bind to the U1 snRNP specific peptides denoted 68 K, A and C. Of these, the 68 K peptide seems to be the most prominent RNP antigen recognized by MCTD sera.

Sera from patients with low and high titers of anti-RNP antibodies have been analyzed for the presence of antibodies binding to recombinant antigens. The cDNA coding for the major part of the 68 K protein was cloned, deletion mutants constructed in prokaryotic expression vectors and different sections of the 68 K protein expressed as parts of recombinant fusion proteins. By this technique we have demonstrated the existence of a major antigenic region and in addition at least two other less frequently recognized antigenic parts of the 68 K peptide. Most high and low titer anti-RNP sera only recognized the major region. In addition a few reacted with a central region of the 68 K protein also recognized by a mouse monoclonal anti-RNP antibody. The most aminoterminal region, which is showing partial sequence homology with a mouse retroviral p30 gag protein contained an epitope that was the major antigen recognized by a single serum.

Anti-La antibodies are found in sera from patients with autoimmune disorders, primarily Sjögren's syndrome and systemic lupus erythematosus and serves as a serological marker for the firstmentioned disease. The La antigen is a phosphorylated nucleoprotein that binds a heterogeneous group of small RNAs, primarily immature pol III transcripts but also some virally encoded RNAs. The molecular weight is estimated to between 45 and 50 kD. Interest in this protein derives both from its role in the processing of pol III transcripts and from its role as an autoantigen. Spontaneously occurring autoantibodies to La have been used as reagents to isolate and characterize the La protein. Identification of the parts of the molecule recognized by the anti-La antibodies may lead to better diagnostic reagents and insights into mechanisms underlying autoimmunity.

In order to study the antigenic properties of the La protein we have isolated a 1650 base pair (bp) long human cDNA encoding an anti-La reactive protein. Restriction enzyme analysis and DNA sequencing was used to compare this clone with two pulished but inconsistent partial sequences. Our clone extends about 220 bp further towards the 5' end and includes a putative initiation codon. The La cDNA was cloned into the pEX 2 expression vector and two deletion clones were made using compatible restriction sites in the insert and the vector. The first subclone contains 740 bp from the 5' end of the La cDNA. The second subclone carries a 400 bp 5' end insert. Stable fusion proteins were obtained both from the initial clone and from the two deletion clones. The recombinant proteins were tested by immunoblotting against a panel of anti-La sera. All reacted with the fusion protein produced by the 1650 bp clone. About half of the anti-La sera showed reactivity against the recombinant protein from the shortest deletion clone. This indicates that in addition to an carboxyterminal epitope, some anti-La sera bind to an epitope on the aminoterminal part of the protein.

A Common RNA Recognition Motif Identified Within a Defined U1 RNA-Binding Domain of the 70 K U1 snRNP Autoantigen

C. C. Query, R. C. Bentley, and J. D. Keene

Department of Microbiology and Immunology, Duke University Medical Center, Durham, NC 27710, USA

The 70 K U1 RNA-associated protein is a component of the U1 small nuclear ribonucleoprotein (snRNP) complex and a major antigen in autoimmune diseases. We have previously demonstrated that the 70 K protein sequence contains similarity in a region of 23 residues to murine leukemia virus (MuLV) group specific antigen $p30^{gag}$. The similarity resides in an antigenic portion of the 70 K protein and is defined by a core consensus sequence, ETPEEREERRR, which occurs as a tandem repeat in $p30^{gag}$ of most mammalian type-C retroviruses. Anti-$p30^{gag}$ antibodies recognized the recombinant 70 K-LacZ fusion protein as well as U1 snRNPs. Using synthetic peptides as competitors, we demonstrated that the region of sequence similarity encompasses the site of immunological cross-reactivity. Thus, autoantibodies reactive with U1 snRNPs were elicited by immunization with retroviral $p30^{gag}$. Based upon these findings, we suggest a role for retroviruses in a model for the initiation of autoimmunity.

Several snRNPs have been implicated in the removal of intervening sequences during precursor messenger RNA splicing. The U1 snRNP, in particular, has been shown to interact with the 5' splice site, at least in part, by base pairing of this site with the 5' terminal 10 nucleotides (nt) of U1 RNA. The human U1 snRNP is composed of the 165 nt U1 RNA and two classes of proteins: U1-specific proteins, 70 K, A, and C; and the Sm complex, consisting of six U snRNP-common proteins. Although these proteins probably play important structural roles in snRNPs and are required for the interaction of U1 snRNP with 5' splice sites, none have been assigned specific functions.

The U1 snRNP-70 K protein has two potential regions of interaction with other structures: the U1 RNA-binding domain (QUERY et al., 1989, Cell **57**, 89−101) and a highly charged arginine-rich RD/RE/RS motif that is present in several proteins which regulate alternative splicing as well as in the retrovirus *gag* protein. This latter region is implicated in *trans-active* regulation of pre-mRNA splice site selection. To investigate the RNA and protein components involved in the specific RNA-protein interaction, we have investigated the recognition properties of the 70 K protein and RNA. *In vitro* translated 70 K protein and 70 K-LacZ fusion protein selectively bound U1 RNA from the total HeLa RNA and also bound U1 transcripts synthesized *in vitro*. Thus, we were able to reconstitute *in vitro* a specific 70 K-U1 RNA complex and demonstrated that the 70 K protein binds directly to U1 RNA.

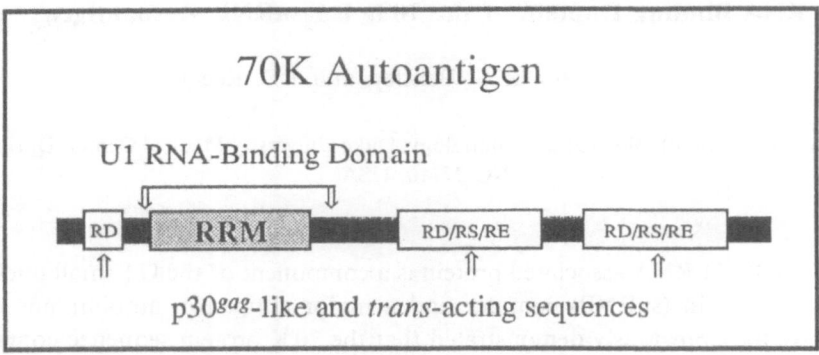

Using *in vitro* translated 70 K deletion mutants and deletion mutants of the 70 K-LacZ fusion protein, we defined the RNA-binding domain of the 70 K protein to a region of 111 amino acids. This domain encompasses an octamer sequence (DREYFUSS et al., 1988, TIBS **13**, 86−91) which has been observed in other proteins associated with RNA but which has not previously been shown to bind directly to a specific RNA sequence. Within the U1 RNA-binding domain, an 80 amino acid consensus sequence was discerned that is conserved in many presumed RNA-binding proteins. This sequence pattern appears to represent an RNA recognition motif (RRM) characteristic of a distinct class to proteins. In addition, this motif may represent a structure common to autoantigens.

To investigate if separable regions within the RNA-binding domain of the 70 K protein are involved in general RNA affinity versus specific RNA binding and which amino acids participate in these interactions, we have isolated point mutants across the 80 amino acid RRM. These mutations have resulted in several phenotypes which indicate important sites of RNA recognition: U 1 RNA-specific binding with altered efficiencies, non-specific RNA-binding, and loss of RNA-binding activity.

Using deletion mutants of U 1 RNA, a region required for binding the 70 K protein was localized. Various RNA fragments were used which delimited the U 1 RNA-binding site to nucleotides 19 – 49 from the 5' cap. Thus, we have determined that a domain of 111 amino acids of the 70 K protein specifically recognizes 31 nucleotides that form a stem-loop structure near the 5' end of U 1 RNA. Currently, we are further characterizing the RNA-binding domain(s) of the 70 K protein and will be investigating possible protein-protein interactions in our efforts to understand the structure and activity of U 1 snRNP in spliceosome complexes.

Characterization of Nucleolar 7-2 RNP Recognized by Sera from Patients with Autoimmune Diseases

R. Reddy, Y. Yuan, and R. Singh

Baylor College of Medicine, Department of Pharmacology, One Baylor Plaza, Houston, Tx 77030, USA

Sera from some patients with autoimmune diseases specifically immuno-precipitate 7-2 RNA-containing ribonucleoprotein particles (3, 5, 6). Three sera, anti-Th (3), To (5) and Wa (6), have been reported to immunoprecipitate 7-2 RNP particles. 7-2 RNA a noncapped small RNA, is also termed RNA M and 7SM RNA. 7-2 RNA, as part of a small ribonucleoprotein particle, is present in the granular compartment of the nucleoli (6).

In this study, the primary sequence of NOVIKOFF hepatoma 7-2 RNA is determined and a possible secondary structure is presented. The NOVIKOFF hepatoma 7-2 RNA is 94% homologous to the recently described mouse mitochondrial RNase MRP RNA suggesting that NOVIKOFF hepatoma 7-2 RNA may be the homologue of mouse MRP RNA. MRP RNase, characterized by CLAYTON and his associates, is a site-specific endoribonuclease involved in primer RNA metabolism in mammalian mitochondria and contains an essential RNA component designated MRP RNA (1, 2, 7). Our results with 7-2 RNA-specific probes also confirm the nucleolar localization of 7-2 RNA reported earlier (4, 6). The presence of 7-2 RNA in nucleoli and in mitochondria suggests that 7-2 RNPs, in addition to being an essential component of mitochondrial RNase, may also be functional in nucleolar RNA processing and ribosome biogenesis. The anti-7-2 RNP antibodies from patients with autoimmune diseases will be helpful in studying the structure and function(s) of 7-2 RNA-containing RNP particles.

References

1. CHANG, D. D. and CLAYTON, D. A. (1987): Science **235**, 1178–1184
2. CHANG, D. D. and CLAYTON, D. A. (1989): Cell **56**, 131–139
3. HASHIMOTO, C. and STEITZ, J. A. (1983): J. Biol. Chem. **258**, 1379–1382
4. REDDY, R. et al. (1981): J. Biol. Chem. **256**, 8452–8457
5. REDDY, R. et al. (1983): J. Biol. Chem. **258**, 1383–1386
6. REIMER, G. et al. (1988): Exp. Cell Res. **176**, 117–128
7. WONG, T. W. and CLAYTON, D. A. (1986): Cell **45**, 817–825

Structure and Antigenicity of the p70 (Ku) Autoantigen

W. H. Reeves, Z. M. Sthoeger, C.-H. Chou, and A. Porges

The Rockefeller University, New York, NY, USA

The Ku (p70/p80) antigen is a macromolecular complex consisting of non-covalently linked ~70 kD and ~80 kD proteins that bind the ends of double-stranded DNA. Autoantibodies to this complex are present in sera of ~1/3 of American patients with SLE, and react with epitopes of both p70 and p80. We have cloned and sequenced cDNAs encoding the p70 protein. The translated amino acid sequence of p70 has a v-myc similarity region, and two leucine repeats, similar in structure to the leucine zipper regions of certain other DNA-binding proteins, that may have a role in p70–p80 dimerization and/or in aligning the DNA-binding domains. By expressing fragments of the human p70 gene in *E. coli*, two antigenic regions were defined, each located near one of the leucine repeats. One of these regions (AA 115–319) reacted weakly, and the other (AA 467–609) strongly, with human autoantibodies. The strongly antigenic region was present on a fusion protein containing the C-terminal 50 residues of p70 (AA 560–609). The corresponding C-terminal regions of murine and canine p70 were unreactive with human autoantibodies, as were the other autoepitopes of p70 and p80. Sequencing of the murine p70 gene and comparison with the human p70 sequence revealed a cluster of sequence differences between amino acids 601 and

609. Deletion of cDNA encoding these residues caused complete unreactivity of the expressed fusion protein with human autoantibodies. Using site-directed mutagenesis, a second region necessary for antigenicity was mapped to AA 560–571. Either human or murine AA 560–571 plus human AA 601–609 were needed for reactivity with the autoantibodies, suggesting that the autoepitope is discontinuous, or that a linear epitope (AA 601–609) is stabilized in some way by AA 560–571. Since human autoantibodies are capable of inhibiting the binding of DNA to Ku (p70/p80), the role of this human-specific C-terminal epitope in DNA binding is under investigation. The significance of the targeting of human-specific sequences by autoantibodies is unclear at present, but such targeting is consistent with the JEMMERSON-MARGOLIASH model of autoreactivity.

Synthetic Peptides an Probes for Autoantibodies

M. H. V. Van Regenmortel, N. Tuaillon, S. Plaué, S. Muller, and J. P. Briand

Laboratoire d'Immunochimie, Institut de Biologie Moléculaire et Cellulaire, CNRS, Strasbourg, France

Many applications of immunochemical research are based on the exploitation of antigenic cross-reactions between proteins and peptides (1). Any linear peptide of 5–10 residues that is found to cross-react with antibodies raised against the corresponding complete protein is labelled a "continuous epitope" of the protein. The peptide may in fact represent only part of a larger discontinuous epitope. Methods have been developed to predict the location of continuous epitopes in the sequence of the protein using a variety of algorithms (2).

Autoantibodies have been shown to bind to a number of intracellular proteins that may or may not represent the immunogenic stimulus. With increasing knowledge of the primary structure of such autoantigens, a number of continuous epitopes have been identified in these molecules. For instance, SLE patients have been found to have autoantibodies that bind an epitope located in the carboxyl-terminal 22 residues for P2 ribosomal protein (3) as well as an epitope corresponding to residues 22–45 of ubiquitin (4). A synthetic 8-residue peptide corresponding to the branched moiety of ubiquinated histone H2A was found to be a particularly good antigenic probe for SLE autoantibodies (5).

Anti-histone antibodies have been detected in sera of patients with rheumatoid arthritis (RA) and juvenile chronic arthritis (JCA). The fine specificity of the autoantibodies was studied with 17 synthetic peptides of the core histones. The peptide 1 – 23 of histone H 3 was recognized by 60% of RA sera and by 62% of JCA sera (6). Many of the sera that did not show any reactivity with the whole histone reacted with various histone peptides. These data indicate that in some cases synthetic peptides may be a superior probe for the detection of autoantibodies than the complete antigen.

References

1. VAN REGENMORTEL, M.H.V. (1987): Antigenic cross-reactivity between proteins and peptides: new insights and applications. Trends Biochem. Sci. **12**, 237 – 240
2. VAN REGENMORTEL, M.H.V., DE MARCILLAC, G. (1988): An assessment of prediction methods in locating continuous epitopes in proteins. Immunol. Lett. **17**, 95 – 108
3. ELKON, K., BONFA, E., LLOVET, R., DANHO, W., WEISSBACH, H., BROT, N. (1988): Properties of the ribosomal P 2 protein autoantigen are similar to those of foreign protein antigens. Proc. Natl. Acad. Sci. USA **85**, 5186 – 5189
4. MULLER, S., BRIAND, J.P., VAN REGENMORTEL, M.H.V. (1988): Presence of antibodies to ubiquitin during the autoimmune response associated with systemic lupus erythematosus. Proc. Natl. Acad. Sci. USA **85**, 8176 – 8180
5. PLAUÉ, S., MULLER, S., VAN REGENMORTEL, M.H.V. (1989): A branched, synthetic octapeptide of ubiquitated histone H 2 A as target of autoantibodies. J. Exp. Med. (in press)
6. TUAILLON, N., MULLER, S., PASQUALI, J.L., BORDIGONI, P., VAN REGENMORTEL, M.H.V. Antibodies from patients with rheumatoid arthritis and juvenile chronic arthritis analyzed with core histone synthetic peptides. (submitted)

cDNA Sequencing and Expression of B/B'-and D-Proteins of RNP Autoantigens in *E. coli*

M. Renz[1], A. Czichos[2], O. Bräunling[1], R. Lührmann[3], H. Giner[1], and H.P. Seelig[2]

[1]DENAGEN Laboratory, Im Neuenheimer Feld 517, 6900 Heidelberg, FRG
[2]Institute for Immunology and experimental Pathology, Kriegsstraße 99, 7500 Karlsruhe, FRG
[3]Institute for Immunology, University of Marburg, 3550 Marburg, FRG

Of the numerous nuclear antigens to which antibodies have been demonstrated in rheumatic diseases, one important group belongs to small nuclear ribonucleoprotein particles (U-sn-RNP). Antibodies to 70 kD-protein epitopes of this particles represent a dominant marker in MCTD, whereas antibodies to the D-protein epitopes may prevail in LE. Other protein epitopes on these particles (A-, B/B′-, C-, E-, F- and G-protein) seem to be of diagnostic value too (1).

We isolated c-DNAs and expressed in *E. coli* the B/B′-, and D-protein of U-sn-RNP and tested their immunoreactivity with patient sera using Western blot and synthetic peptides.

B/B′-protein: Sequence information of the N-terminal peptide of B/B′-protein was used to synthesize oligonucleotides to all codons in order to screen a human pituitary gland lambda gt 10 c-DNA library. In one of the sequenced clones a ATG signal was observed initiating an open reading frame of 720 nucleotides (24.376 kD). Colinearity was observed with the N-terminal peptide as well as with two other tryptic peptides. The most distinguished features of this amino acid sequence are proline-rich motifs close to the C-terminus. Induction of protein synthesis of the expression plasmid lead to the production of a protein which was recognized by anti-Sm sera. 23 sera positive for antibodies reacting with the B/B′-protein in Western blots from HeLa cell nuclear extracts showed strong immunoreactivity with the expressed B/B′-fusion protein. Preliminary results of epitope mapping with B/B′ positive sera tested by Western blot revealed two antigenic regions corresponding to the proline-rich motifs mentioned above.

D-protein: The same library used for isolation of the B/B′-clones was screened with a 29mer mixture of oligonucleotides constructed according to the amino acid sequence of the N-terminal tryptic peptide. The 555 bp long EcoRI insert of one clone was completely sequenced. An open reading frame of 357 bp encoded a protein of 119 amino acids with a calculated molecular weight of 13.282 kD which is in the range of that estimated by SDS-PAGE. The coding region of this clone is identical to a Sm-D-clone publishing during this work was in progress (2). Minor differences exist mainly in the 3′ untranslated region. A recombinant D-protein construct reacted with 8 out of 12 selected sera positive for anti-D with HeLa cell nuclear extract. With the expression of this protein in eucaryotic systems this problem migth be overcome.

The results give us good reasons to hope, that the important marker antigens of this group of rheumatoid diseases may be soon available as fusion proteins or as synthetic peptides suitable for development of diagnostic tests.

References

1. HABETS, W. J., DE ROOIJ, D. J., HOET, M. H., VAN DE PUTTE, L. B., VAN VENROOIJ, W. J. (1985): Quantitation of anti-RNP and anti-SM antibodies in MCTD and SLE patients by immunoblotting. Clin. Exp. Immunol. **59**, 457–466
2. ROKEACH, L. A., HASELBY, J. A., HOCH, S. O. (1988): Molecular cloning of a cDNA encoding the human Sm-D autoantigen, Proc. Natl. Acad. Sci. USA, **85**, 4832–4836

Compartmentalization of Nuclear Antigens Detected by Autoantibodies

N. Ringertz, U. Nyman, M. Bergman, and I. Pettersson

Department of Medical Cell Genetics, Medical Nobel Institute, Karolinska Institutet, Box 60400, 10401 Stockholm, Sweden

Autoantibodies of the Sm and RNP specificities are directed against small nuclear RNA-protein (sRNP) complexes involved in the splicing of RNA polymerase II transcripts. Anti-La antibodies react with another class of RNA-protein complexes carrying the La-antigen, a termination factor in RNA polymerase III transcription. Both the autoantibodies and monoclonal antibodies derived from autoimmune mice have been useful tools in the analysis of RNA splicing and in the study of the functional organization of the interphase nucleus. Another important application has been in the study of the assembly of snRNP complexes and their translocation to the nucleus.

We have used the heterokaryons system to analyze the assembly of snRNP particles in reactivating chick erythrocyte nuclei. Nucleated chick erythrocytes (CE) are terminally differentiated, non-dividing cells. The nuclei (CEn) are transcriptionally inactive, lack nucleoli and have a compact, tightly condensed chromatin. The nuclei of mature erythrocytes are depleted in non-histone proteins and small nuclear RNP-protein (snRNP) complexes. Following Sendai virus induced fusion of CE with transcriptionally active mammalian cells, heterokaryons are formed in which the CEn undergo transcriptional reactivation. Previous studies have shown that a number of mammalian nuclear proteins enter the CEn compartment. The present investigation examines if CE nuclei accumulate snRNP complexes as part of the reactivation process that takes place in heterokaryons. Furthermore, efforts are made to determine if the snRNP complexes were of chick or rat origin and if their appearance depended on transcription of chick or rat genes.

We examined CE nuclei in heterokaryons for the expression of four snRNP related nuclear antigens (Sm, RNP, F78 and M3G-cap) and for the La antigen. Inactive erythrocyte nuclei showed very low levels of expression of snRNP and La antigens. During reactivation in rat myoblast heterokaryons the expression of these antigens increased but with different kinetics for different antigens. Blocking of chick transcription did not block the appearance of Sm, RNP, cap, and La antigens, but did effectively inhibit expression of the F78 antigen. The latter antigen has previously been shown to be present on high molecular complexes of snRNP particles rather than on individual snRNP particles. The results also suggest that *rat* snRNP proteins are imported into the *chick* nuclei and that, with the possible exception of the F78 antigen, this translocation is independent of chick RNA synthesis. In addition, the data suggest that accumulation of snRNP complexes in the chick erythrocyte nuclei is parallelled by a depletion of the rat myoblast nuclei in such complexes.

Anti-A. R.: A New Autoantibody/ies in Autoimmune Chronic Active Hepatitis (CAH) that Precipitates a 4.5 S RNA

J. L. Rodriguez-Sanchez, P. Asunción, M. Catalfamo, C. Gelpi, C. Juarez, Ma. J. Amengual

Hospital de la Santa Creu i Sant Pau, Hospital Universitari de la Facultat de Medicina de la Universitat Autónoma de Barcelona, San Antonio Ma. Claret 167, 08025 Barcelona, Spain

A new autoantibody/ies was detected in the serum of three patients with CAH. The antibody/ies precipitated a small RNA running slighly slower than most tRNAs. Immunoprecipitation of ^{35}S-methionine labelled Friend leukemia cell extracts with the patient sera and analysis by SDS-PAGE, also showed precipitation of two polypeptides of 57 and 58 kDa. Neither 4.5S RNA, nor 57–58 kDa polypeptides were precipitated by the sera of other 44 patients with CAH by the 220 tested sera from patients with various hepatic and non-hepatic disorders (21 primary biliary cirrhosis, 14 acute viral hepatitis, 10 non-A non-B hepatitis, 16 HIV+, 46 LES, 10 PM, 23 PSS, 15 primary SS, 50 RA, 10 MCTD and 30 NHS).

The three positive patients had the following clinical characteristics in common: They were young woman, with amenorrhea, hepatic lessions and showed poor response to immunosuppressive therapy. One of these patients had hypergammaglobulinemia.

Other autoantibodies detected by indirect immunofluorescence are summarized in Table 1.

Table 1. Autoantibodies in anti-4.5 S RNA positive ACAH Patients

Patient	ANA	SMA	AMA	LMA	LCA	Cyt A	LKM
1	Hw	−	−	+	−	+ +	−
2	Hw, M+ +	−	−	+	−	−	−
3	H+ + +	+ + +	−	−	−	+ +	−

ANA, antinuclear antibodies; *SMA*, smooth muscle antibodies; *AMA*, antimitochondrial antibodies; *LMA*, liver membrane antibodies; *LCA*, liver cytoplasmic antibodies; *Cyt A*, cytoskeletal antibodies. IIF on Hep-2 cells

The presence of anti-A. R. antibodies, different from the antiactine, anti-LKM, and anti-SLA antibodies described to date, could be a new marker for a subgroup of CAH.

Immunological Crossreactivity Between RNA Polymerase I and the Glycine Rich Repeats of Epstein-Barr Virus Nuclear Antigen

K. Rose and G. Rhodes

University of Texas Medical School, Houston, Texas, USA, and Scripps Clinic and Research Foundation, La Jolla, California, USA

Antibodies were raised against synthetic peptides corresponding to amino acid sequences found within or near the glycine-rich repeating region of the Epstein-Barr viral nuclear antigen, EBNA. These antibodies, but not those raised against other regions of the EBV genome, were able to bind to the DNA-dependent enzyme RNA polymerase I and to inhibit RNA synthesis in vitro. Antibodies against the synthetic EBNA peptides bound to the 65-kDa polypeptide associated with the polymerase. Polyclonal antibodies raised against purified RNA polymerase I itself were capable of binding to the synthetic peptides corresponding to the repeat regions but not to other regions of the EBV genome. These data indicate that RNA polymerase I and EBNA contain common antigenic determinants and suggest that autoantibodies reactive with this polymerase may have a viral etiology.

Drug Induced Anti-Histone Antibodies Reflect Nucleosomal Substructures

R. L. Rubin and R. W. Burlingame

Research Institute of Scripps Clinic, La Jolla California, USA

Anti-histone antibodies commonly arise as a side effect of therapy with a variety of drugs. Previous attempts to define the specificity of these autoantibodies were largely confined to studies with individual histones and their fragments. Since histones normally exist as oligomeric complexes with DNA, we examined the binding of drug-induced antibodies to native nucleohistone and its component subunits.

Two distinct patterns of reactivity were observed. One pattern was centered around the antigenicity of (H2A−H2B)-containing structures, especially when complexed to DNA, such as the (H2A−H2B)-DNA subnucleosome particle, H1-stripped chromatin and trypsinized H1-stripped chromatin. Sera showing this reactivity failed to bind (H3−H4)$_2$-containing complexes or DNA. The other pattern had essentially the converse characteristics in that the antibodies reacted most strongly with native H2A−H2B dimers, H3−H4 tetramers and H1 when these particles were not complexed to DNA. H1-stripped chromatin was largely non-reactive, and these sera showed only weak antinuclear antibody staining properties. These two patterns of reactivity were independent of serum concentration, and quantitative determination of protein and DNA in the ELISA wells used for antibody determination and other controls demonstrated that these results could not be explained by any significant assay bias.

The H2A−H2B based antibody reactivity displayed a remarkable association with symptomatic drug-induced lupus. All 21 patients with a lupus-like illness induced by procainamide and 7 patients with quinidine-induced lupus with anti-histone antibodies had IgG antibodies displaying strongest reactivity with the (H2A−H2B)-DNA complex and showed little reactivity with (H3−H4)$_2$-DNA in any form. Of 24 patients with procainamide-induced anti-histone antibodies without symptoms, only 5 displayed enhanced reactivity with (H2A−H2B)-DNA complex, and two of these patients went on to develop symptomatic disease. Thus, IgG antibodies to the (H2A−H2B)-DNA complex is diagnostic of procainamide and quinidine-induced lupus and may antedate the appearance of distinct symptoms. We have also found these antibodies in patients with lupus induced by other drugs such as acebutalol, a-methyldopa and penicillamine.

The pattern of reactivity with DNA-free histones was observed in 18/19 sera from patients treated with chlorpromazine and 14/17 patients with hydralazine-induced lupus. These were predominantly IgM antibodies and the highest reactivity was directed against H1, followed by the (H3−H4)$_2$ tetramer and the H2A−H2B dimer. Many of these sera had antibodies to denatured DNA, but DNA inhibited binding of anti-histone antibodies to the native histone-histone complexes and to H1.

Normally, a mechanism presumably exists for suppressing autoimmunity to chromatin substructures, and we suggest that anti-histone antibody-inducing drugs interfere with autoimmune tolerance. Antibodies induced by hydralazine or chlorpromazine may be elicited by immunogenic forms of DNA-free histones in a milieu of active tolerization by mononucleosomes. In contrast, antibodies in patients with procainamide-induced lupus may be elicited by partially proteolyzed chromatin, but suppression of immune response to epitopes not contained within (H2A−H2B)-DNA complexes could be explained by tolerogenic forms of the (H3−H4)$_2$-DNA tetramer. Such epitope restriction is supported by coblocking studies in which antibodies from procainamide-induced lupus sera failed to inhibit antibodies induced by chlorpromazine from binding to the H2A−H2B dimer. Precise definition of these epitopes may require analysis at the 3° and 4° structural levels.

Anti-histone antibody-inducing drugs have diverse chemical structure, but may be metabolized into products with similar properties. The present studies demonstrating that these antibodies display a straighforward relationship to chromatin structure suggest that drug metabolites may break immune tolerance by disturbing normal pathways of chromatin degradation.

Epitope Mapping of the Ro-RNP Autoantigen Using Recombinant Polypeptides

M. R. Saitta, S. L. Deutscher, F. C. Arnett, and J. D. Keene

Duke University Medical Center, Durham, NC and UTHSC, Houston, Tx, USA

Autoantibodies against the Ro ribonucleoprotein complex (Ro-RNP) occur frequently in the sera of patients with autoimmune connective tissue disease (ACTD), but the significance of the epitopes recognized by these responses remains unknown. We have successfully engineered, from the full-lenght cDNA clone, a series of site-directed cDNA constructs of the human Ro-RNP 60 k protein. Polypeptides generated by *in vitro* transcription and translation of these partial templates were used in immunoprecipitation (IP) experiments to define regions of the 60 k antigen reactive with Ro autoantibodies. The recombinant peptides reacted with polyclonal rabbit anti-Ro serum but not with normal human serum.

Sera from patients with the anti-Ro specificity and ACTD were tested for their ability to immunoprecipitate the recombinant Ro peptides. Epitopes were identified along the entire length of the Ro 60 k protein and several different patterns of reactivity were observed. Data to date using sera from twelve patients shows no striking associations between the pattern of epitope reactivity and clinical diagnosis, the presence of La autoantibodies, or HLA-DR/DQ genotype. IP using a range of concentrations of antisera suggest that the reactivity profiles reflect quantitatively different antibody titers to specific epitopes. Further experiments using in vivo expressed polypeptides in a solid-phase assay are in progress.

Idiotype Network and Anti-DNA Antibody Production

T. Sasaki, S. Shibata, N. Harata, E. Tamate, and K. Yoshinaga

The Second Department of Internal Medicine, Tohoku University School of Medicine, Sendai, Japan

It has not been well known as to whether the production of autoantibodies is regulated through idiotype network system for self tolerance mechanism. We obtained murine monoclonal anti-idiotypic antibody (Ab 2, D1 E2) directed to paratope of human monoclonal anti-ssDNA antibody, 0−81. The administration of D1 E2 caused profound suppression of anti-ssDNA responses in Balb/c mice or $NZB/W\,F_1$ mice. The serial administration of D1 E2 conjugated with cytotoxic agent (neocarzinostatin, NCS) brought into a prolonged survival and a decreased anti-DNA autoantibody production in female NZB/W F_1 mice. Then, we developed murine hybridoma producing anti-D1 E2 antibody (Ab 3, ET-1). ET-1 specifically blocked the binding of D1 E2 to 0−81. The pretreatment with ET-1-conjugated with NCS evoked an enhanced anti-ssDNA responses to aligonucleotide-KLE stimulation in nonautoimmune mice, where the numbers of 0−81 idiotype-positive cells were significantly increased. These results indicate that idiotype network mechanism may be closely associated with anti-DNA antibody production in vivo.

In Vitro Binding of A and B″ snRNP Proteins to U1 and U2 snRNAs

D. Scherly[1], W. C. Boelens[2], I. W. Mattaj[1], and W. J. van Venrooij[2]

[1] EMBL, Heidelberg, FRG
[2] Department of Biochemistry, Nijmegen, Holland

In addition to the Sm proteins common to U1, U2, U5 and U4/U6 snRNP particles, U1 snRNP contains three specific proteins called 70 K, A and C; two others, called A′ and B″, are specific for U2 snRNPs. Using cDNAs coding for the human A and B″ proteins (P. T. G. SILLEKENS et al. (1987): EMBO J. **6**, 3841−3848; W. J. HABETS et al. (1987): PNAS **84**, 2421−2445) we have produced *in vitro* the corresponding proteins and have analysed their binding to U1 and U2 snRNAs *in vitro*.

In a first step we have used mutant U snRNAs transcripts to define their RNA binding sites. These sites show striking sequence similarities. It has already been reported that the amino acid sequence of A and B″ are very similar. Nevertheless, A and B″ bind both *in vitro* and *in vivo* specifically to their respective U snRNAs.

In vitro mutagenesis of the A and B″ cDNAs is being used to analyse the determinants of binding specificity and affinity.

Expression of the 70 kD RNP Autoantigen in *E. coli* and Its Use in ELISA-Screening of Patients Sera

H. P. Seelig[1], C. Heim[2], C. Wieland[1], M. Renz[2]

[1] Private Institute for Immunology and Experimental Pathology, Kriegsstraße 99,
D-7500 Karlsruhe, FRG
[2] DENAGEN Laboratory, Im Neuenheimer Feld 517, D-6900 Heidelberg, FRG

Of the numerous nuclear antigens to which antibodies have been demonstrated in rheumatic diseases, one important group belongs to small nuclear ribonucleoprotein particles (U-sn-RNP). Antibodies to 70 kD-protein epitopes of this particles represent a dominant marker in MCTD (1). We expressed in *E. coli* the 70 kD-protein of U-sn-RNP and developed a specific and sensitive ELISA test for antibody screening in patient sera.

An insert of 1293 bp of the c-DNA encoding 87% of the 70 kD-protein was subcloned into pEMBL vector and ligated into the expression vector pEX 34 b (2), which was transferred into *E. coli* 537 containing a temperature sensitive mutant of the λ repressor gene cI on a kanamycin resistant plasmid (pcI 857) (3). The fusion protein was purified by DEAE column chromatography (linear NaCl gradient, 5 M urea, 10 mM Tris-HCl pH 7.4). Fractions between 350 and 550 mM NaCl contained essentially pure 70 kD fusion protein components as judged by SDS-PAGE and immunoblotting. Using microtiterplates coated with purified fusion protein (0.7 μg/ml, carbonat buffer pH 9.5) 799 sera were tested in a sandwich ELISA and compared with the results using RNase digested and nondigested calf thymus extract (CTE) as coating material.

None of the control sera (N = 654) which were negative with CTE showed antibodies reacting with the 70 kD-protein (Table). There is a high percentage of sera positive with RNase digested and non-digested CTE, but not reacting with the 70 kD-protein (N = 76). About 50% of these sera revealed antibodies reacting with Sm-antigen (B/B′- and D-protein) and/or A- and C-proteins as could be shown on Western blots. The remaining anti-Sm negative sera of this group reacted with several non characterized proteins in Western blots. 33 sera reacting with the 70 kD-protein as well as with the native and RNase-digested CTE could be classified to contain anti-RNP and anti-Sm activity, 36 sera reacting with native CTE and with the 70 kD-protein could be classified as true anti-RNP. The use of the 70 kD-protein as antigen may fullfill the requirements of a simple and specific test for RNP-antibodies found in patients with MCTD and LE. A negative test with the 70 kD-protein may exclude the diagnosis of MCTD.

Table 1. Results of EELISA test using 70 kD-protein antigen and RNase digested and non-digested calf thymus nuclear extract (CTE, precipitated with $30\% - 60\%$ $(NH_4)_2SO_4$). CTE showed no reactivity with anti-SS-A, -SS-B, -Scl-70, -histones, -ds-DNA, -ss-DNA. Anti-Sm were reactive with the digested and non-digested CTE, anti-RNP sera with un-digested CTE

Sera N	No. of positive results			
	CTE	CTE RNase	70 kD-protein	Classification
654	0	0	0	no antibodies
76	76	76	0	others/anti-Sm
33	33	33	33	anti-Sm/RNP
36	36	0	36	anti-RNP

References

1. HABETS, W. J., DE ROOIJ, D. J., HOET, M. H., VAN DE PUTTE, L. B. VAN VENROOIJ, W. J. (1985): Quantitation of anti-RNP and anti-SM antibodies in MCTD and SLE patients by immunoblotting. Clin. Exp. Immunol. **59**, 457–466
2. THEISSEN, H., ETZERODT, M., REUTER, R., SCHNEIDER, C., LOTTSPEICH, F., ARGOS, P., LÜHRMANN, R., PHILIPSON, L. (1986): Cloning of the human cDNA for the U1 RNA-associated 70 K protein. EMBO Journal **5**, 3209–3217
3. REMAUT, E., STANSSENS, P., FIERS, W. (1986): Plasmid vectors for high-efficiency expression controlled by the PL promotor of coliphage lambda, Gene **15**, 81–93

The Autoantibody Expresion in Cultured Cell Lines of Human Keratinocytes Transformed by Virus and by Ultraviolet Light in SLE and Other Autoimmune Diseases

J. Sequi[1], I. Leigh[2], and D. A. Isenberg[3]

[1]Immunology Department, Ramon y Cajal Hospital, Madrid, Spain
[2]Department of Dermatology, London Hospital, London, Great Britain
[3]Bloomsbury Rheumatology Unit, University College and Middlesex Hospital Medical School, London, Great Britain

Summary: The Antinuclear Antibodies are one of the criteria accepted by the ARA, in the revision of the classification of SLE. The objetive of the present work is to study the expresion of the nuclear and cytoplasmic antigens, in cell lines transformed by virus and by ultraviolet light, taking into account the existance of differences among several diseases and the type and grade of the activity of SLE (1).

Material: Forty patients with SLE have been studied, with samples in active and inactive phase, classified in groups of eight by the first expression of the illness in: 1) Renal disease, 2) central nervous system involvement, 3) joint and skin disease only, 4) pleuropericardial symptoms and 5) a group with recurrent thrombosis and/or spontaneous abortion and thrombocytopenia accompanied by anticardiolipin antibodies (2). As disease controls sera from ten patients each with rheumatoid arthritis, primary Sjogren's syndrome, adult onset myositis and scleroderma; and 20 serum samples controls.

Method: The expression of autoantibodies, was studied using the Indirect Immunofluorescent technique, with cell lines kept in culture of:

1. Hep-2 cells.
2. SVK-14 cells, Human Keratinocytes transformed by virus.
3. UVK-cells, Human Keratinocytes transformed by ultraviolet light.
4. Human Keratinocytes.
5. Human Keratinocytes exposed to the ultraviolet ligth.

Results:

1. The expression of autoantibody is larger in patients with SLE, than in other group studied.
2. The intensity of the staining is larger in cell lines transformed by ultraviolet light (UVK-cell), than in the cell lines transformed by virus (SVK-14-cell).
3. A change in the histological expression is observed in the staining of the antigens, showing nuclear staining in SVK-cell, while the serum in cell transformed by ultraviolet light change to staining the nuclear membrane or the cytoplas-

mic antigens. This may, of course, reflect alterations in antigenicity brought about by ultraviolet radiation.

References

1. TAN, E. M., COHEN, A. S., FRIES, J. F. et al. (1984): The 1982 revised criteria for the classification of systemic lupus erythematosus. Arthritis Rheum. **27**, 125–138
2. TAN, E. M., CHAN, E. K. L., SULLIVAN, K. F., RUBIN, R. L. (1988): Antinuclear antibodies (ANAs): Diagnostically specific immune markers and dues to want the understanding of systemic autoimmunity. Clin. Immunol. Immunopathol. **47**, 121–141

The B Cell Activation in Autoimmunity

T. Shirai, K. Hasegawa, M. Abe, T. Okada, S. Hirose, and H. Sato

Department of Pathology, Juntendo University School of Medicine, 2-1-1 Hongo, Bunkyo-ku, Tokyo 113, Japan

Unlike splenic B cells from normal BALB/c mice, those from autoimmune-prone NZB×NZW (B/W)F1 young mice were hyperresponsive to interleukin 2 (IL 2) and proliferated even in the absence of prior stimulation signals. We found that the B cell subpopulation responsible for this event belongs to that with 6B2 (B220)-dull, Ly1 (CD5)-positive phenotypes. Cell cycle analysis revealed that the 6B2-dull, Ly1 B cell subpopulation contains a significant number of cells at phases of G1A and G1B, while the majority of 6B2-bright B cells belongs to G0. It appears, therefore, that most of the Ly1 B cells in young B/W F1 mice are already stimulated *in vivo* to the stage of early activation, so that they respond to IL 2 without prior stimuli. However, the B/W F1 mice showed a rapid decrease in the proportion of splenic Ly1 B cells, beginning at about 6 months of age. This was associated with the hyporesponsiveness to IL 2 of splenic B cells. While the related mechanisms are not well understood, there are at least 2 possibilities: First, the Ly1 B lineage cells disappear in B/W F1 mice with aging. Alternatively, as the process of activation and differentiation advances in these cells, they lose the phenotype of Ly1. The latter possibility will be discussed in relation to isotype switch of Ly1 B lineage cells.

Rheumatoid Factor Idiotypes in Lymphoproliferative Disorders in Patients with SJÖGREN's Syndrome

S. Sugai, S. Shimizu, J. Tachibana, M. Sawada, and S. Konda

Division of Hematology and Immunology, Department of Internal Medicine, Kanazawa Medical University, Uchinada-machl, Kahoku-gun, Ishikawa 920-02, Japan

SJÖGREN's syndrome (SS) is an autoimmune disease characterized by autoantibody production and lymphoproliferation in salivary and lacrymal glands and in other extraglandular sites. SS patients have a high titer of rheumatoid factor (RF) and sometimes develope lymphoproliferative disorders such as monoclonal gammopathy and malignant lymphoma. In order to study the relationship between SS and lymphoproliferative disorders, we examined RF idiotypes in serum monoclonal immunoglobulins (Ig) and in the cell surface and cytoplasmic Igs of lymphoma cells in patients with SS.

Patients and Methods

Serum monoclonal Igs were studied in 22 patients with SS, 8 with WALDEN-STRÖM's macroglobulinemia (WM), 14 with multiple myeloma (MM) and 4 with monoclonal Ig-producing lymphomas. Lymphoma cells of the B cell type in 4 SS patients and another 22 patients were studied.

Four monoclonal anti-idiotypic antibodies were produced against antigen-binding sites of RFs by immunizing 4 monoclonal RFs derived from 3 patients with SS (IgM-K, IgA-L and IgA-K) and one patient with WM (IgM-K).

Cross-reactive idiotypes (CRI) of monoclonal Igs were examined by ELISA and the immunoblotting technique done by agarose gel electrophoresis, isoelectric focusing and SDS-PAGE. Reverse immunoblotting was also done by the reaction between idiotype determinants on electrophoresis plates and anti-idiotype antibodies coupled to nitrocellulose membranes.

Cell surface Igs and idiotpye were stained by the immunofluorescent method. The ABC immunoperoxidase technique was used for cytoplasmic Igs and idiotypes.

Results and Discussion

(1) By immunoblotting of agarose gel electrophoresis and SDS-PAGE, CRI of RFs were detected not only in monoclonal RFs but also in non-RF monoclonal Igs, and even in monoclonal Igs with different heavy- or light chains from the original RFs used for immunization. CRI were found in 58% to 92% monoclonal

Igs in 22 patients with SS. These incidences were higher than those (30% − 37%) of monoclonal Igs in patients with MM, WM or ML. These data were confirmed by the results obtained by ELISA.

(2) Cell surface Igs and idiotypes as well as cytoplasmic Igs and idiotypes were examined in 4 lymphomas in SS patients and in 22 lymphomas in other patients. CRI of RFs were found in one to 3 SS patients, but only two out of other 22 patients showed RF idiotypes.

Our results show that monoclonal Igs in the serum and in the lymphoma cells in patients with SS have RF idiotypes more frequently than those in other B cell malignancies without any evidence of autoimmune disorders, indicating that monoclonal proliferation in SS patients, benign or malignant, frequently takes place in RF-producing clones.

Snurps and Scyrps − Insights into the Biology of RNA Processing

J. A. Steitz

Department of Molecular Biophysics and Biochemistry, Howard Hughes Medical Institute, Yale University School of Medicine, New Haven, CT 06510, USA

The most abundant snRNPs in mammalian cells are those involved in splicing. However, there exist many low abundance snRNPs of the same (Sm) class. These include the U7 snRNP, which is required for histone mRNA 3' end maturation, and other particles that potentially participate in polyadenylation or other pre-mRNA processing events. Work with R. DESROSIERS' lab (New England Primate Center, Harvard) has revealed that five small RNAs encoded by *Herpesvirus saimiri* become incorporated into Sm snRNPs; three of these exhibit perfect complementarity to the hexanucleotide polyadenylation signal as well as homology to mRNA destabilization sequences. Whether they are involved in polyadenylation or in mRNA stabilization in transformed T cells is currently under investigation. Collaborative studies with K. VAN DOREN and D. HIRSH (Synergen) previously demonstrated that spliced leader transcripts involved in trans-splicing in both nematodes and typanosomes associate with Sm proteins. The structures of these spliced leader (SL) RNAs suggest that they may fulfill a dual function − serving as both 5' exon and U 1 snRNP − in the trans-splicing reaction. Evidence supporting the idea that SL RNAs activate their own 5' splice sites will be discussed.

A new subset of mammalian snRNPs distinct from the Sm particles has recently been identified. These are localized in the nucleolus and contain a shared autoantigen (fibrillarin). Analyses of the U3, U8, and U13 RNAs reveal a common sequence which may comprise the fibrillarin binding site. Potential functions of these particles in ribosome biogenesis will be considered.

Genetic Restriction of Autoantibody Production in Patients with Systemic Lupus Erythematosus

H. A. F. Stephens[1], D. Isenberg[2], P. J. Maddison[3], K. I. Welsh[1], and G. S. Panayi[1]

[1] Molecular Immunogenetics Laboratory, Guy's Hospital, London, Great Britain
[2] UCH/Middlesex Hospital, London, Great Britain
[3] Royal National Hospital for Rheumatic Diseases, Bath, Great Britain

Systemic lupus erythematosus (SLE) the prototype non-organ specific or systemic autoimmune disease, is characterised by immune response to a wide range of autoantigens leading to a progressively destructive vasculitis. Serological abnormalities include antibodies to the ribonucleoproteins (RNPs) Ro, La, Sm, and U1 RNP. The presence of one or more of these anti-RNP antibodies tends to associate with certain clinical features, suggesting they play a role in the pathogenesis of the disease.

Genetic predisposition to SLE has been associated with several alleles of the MHC. Associations most commonly reported have been with HLA B8, DR3, DR2, and DQw2, as well as the null alleles of the second and fourth components of complement. When autoantibody subsets of SLE are considered certain HLA antigen associations become stronger. For example DR3 and/or DR2 are found in patients producing anti-Ro and anti-La, while DR4 has been associated with anti-U1 RNP. Thus class II control, either qualitative or quantitative, has been implicated in influencing the pathogenesis of SLE. However conventional HLA class II typing is notoriously difficult and unreliable in SLE patients, largely due to the prevalence of leukopaenia in these patients. As polymorphism of the DR, DQ, and DP loci can now be accurately defined by Southern blot analysis of test DNAs, this technique has been used in our laboratory to re-examine the associations between class II alleles and anti-RNP antibody production in SLE patients.

To date 38 patients with known autoantibody profiles to either Ro, Ro and La, or U1 RNP and/or Sm have been analysed. DNA prepared from these patients was genotyped with 5 class II locus and chain-specific probes, namely DR-β (DRB1), DQ-α (DQA1), DQ-β (DQB1) DP-α (DPA1), and DP-β (DPB1). By analysing the class II restriction fragment length polymorphism (RFLP) patterns in these patients, three major associations were observed (Table 1). 14/16 anti-Ro producers shared DQA RFLPs associated with all variants of DQw1. 10/11 anti-Ro/La producers demonstrated DRB, DQA, and DQB RFLP patterns associated with DR3. 12/12 anti-U1 RNP/Sm producers demonstrated DQB RFLP patterns associated with all variants of DQw3. These data confirm the association between DR3 and anti-Ro/La production, but redefine associations between class II alleles and the production of antibodies to Ro, U1 RNP, and Sm. As yet no obvious correlations between DPA or DPB genotypes and anti-RNP antibody profiles can be detected.

Together the primary associations between recognised HLA genotypes and autoantibody profiles in SLE patients, suggest that responses to distinct RNPs are genetically restricted by allelic products of the HLA class II region. From the above associations we would predict that presentation of an immunogenic peptide derived from the Ro antigen, is primarily restricted by a preferential interaction with an epitope unique to the DQA1 chain of all variants of the DQw1 allele. The third hypervariable (HV) region of the first protein domain (positions 45–54) of the DQA1 chain of all variants of DQw1 is identical, and differs significantly from the equivalent region of all variants of DQw2 and DQw3. Similarly, presentation of another peptide on the Ro molecule, and a peptide on the La antigen, are restricted by preferential interactions with epitopes unique to the DRB1 chain of DR3. These epitopes could be located in the second or third HV regions (positions 25–35, and 71–80 respectively), of the DRB1 chain of DR3, which differ from equivalent regions in all other DR alleles. Finally, presentation of peptides derived from the Sm and U1 RNP molecules, are primarily restricted by preferential interactions with an epitope conserved in the DQB1 chain of all variants of DQw3 (the third HV region, positions 66–77).

Table 1. Major HLA class II genotype associations with anti-RNP antibody profiles in SLE patients

		DQA1 (DQw1)	DRB1 (DR3)	DQB1 (DQw3)
Anti-Ro	(n = 16)	14 (86%)	6	10
Anti-Ro/La	(n = 11)	4	10 (91%)	6
Anti-Sm/U1 RNP	(n = 12)	8	2	12 (100%)

Localization of an Immunopathologically Important Epitope in the Bovine Retinal S-Antigen by the Pepscan Method

R. Stiemer[1], H. Gausepohl[2], M. Mirshahi[1], Y. de Kozak[1], M. Kraft[2], J. P. Faure[1], and R. Frank[2]

[1]Laboratoire d'Immunopathologie de l'Oeil, INSERM U 86, Paris, France
[2]European Molecular Biology Laboratory, Heidelberg, FRG

S-antigen (48 k Da protein or arrestin), a soluble protein of retinal photoreceptors, was studied for its autoantigenic properties in the induction of experimental autoimmune uveoretinitis (EAU) (1) and for its function in the visual transduc-

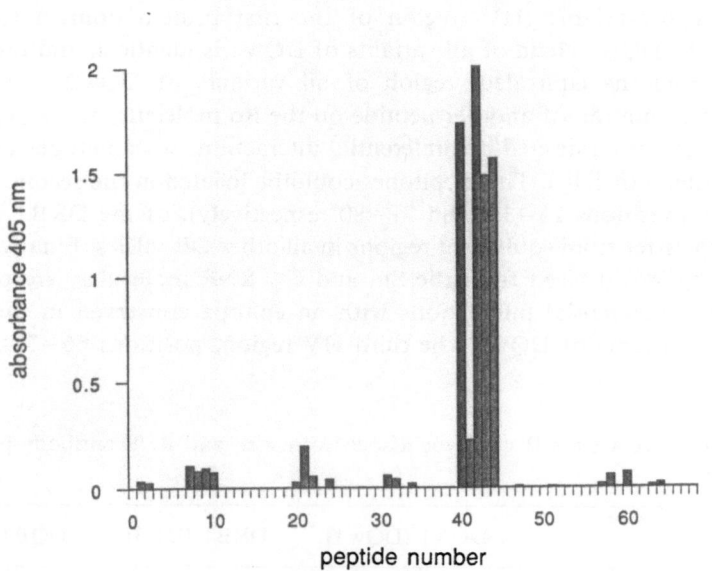

Fig. 1. a Immunoreactivity of S-Ag N-terminal peptides 1 – 68 using 10 µg/ml protein A purified mab S2D2. **b** Titration ELISA of protein A purified mab S2D2, serially diluted starting with 10 mg/ml, on S-antigen (0.01 nM/well) or S-antigen peptide S2 (1 nM/well). **c** Competition ELISA using fixed concentration of affinity purified mab S2D2 (0.1 pM/well) with four different synthetic peptides, serially diluted starting with the initial concentration of 1000 molar excess of the peptides over the coated S-antigen (0.02 nM/well). S2: EPVDGVVLVDPE (39 – 50), S3: KKIKVLVEQVT (235 – 245), S4: QVTNVVLYSSDY (243 – 254), M: DTNLASSTIIKEGIDKTV (303 – 320). **d** Amino acid replacement experiment with the S-Ag aa 40 – 48, i.e. PVDGVVLVD and the TNF aa 36 – 42, i.e., NGVELRD using protein A purified mab S2D2 at the same concentration

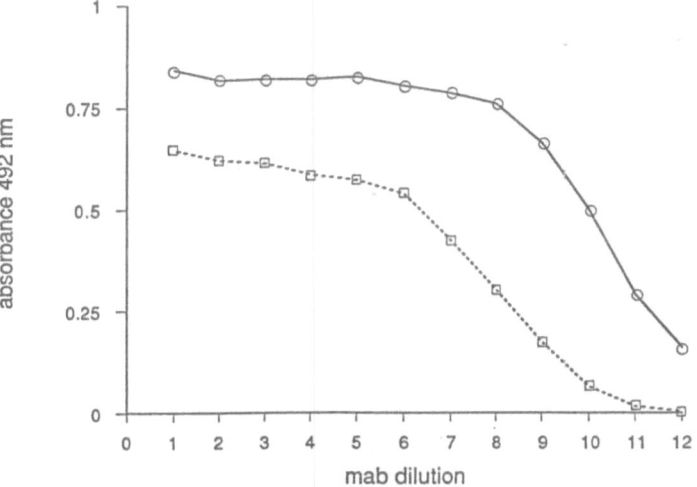

b) —⊖— **S-Ag**
  ⋯⊟⋯ **peptide S2**

Fig. 1b

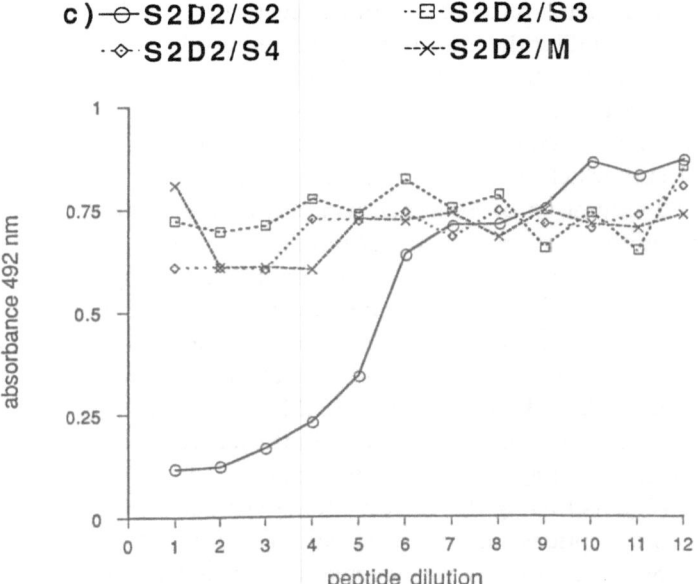

c) —⊖— **S2D2/S2**   ⋯⊟⋯ **S2D2/S3**
  ⋯◇⋯ **S2D2/S4**   —✕— **S2D2/M**

Fig. 1c

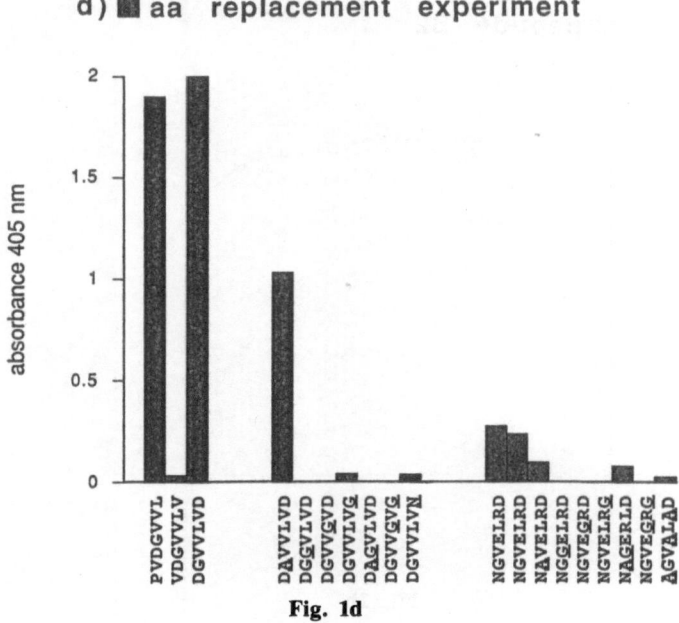

Fig. 1d

tion system (2). The complete amino acid sequence (404 residues) of the protein has been determined in 1987 (3). It was shown that some monoclonal antibodies (mab) against S-antigen, recognizing phylogenetically stable epitopes (4), especially mab S2D2, inhibit the induction of uveoretinitis by simultaneous injection of S-antigen and the mab in an experimental animal system, suggesting an important immunopathological role of the corresponding epitopes (5). The same suppressive effect was achieved by active immunization with the S-antigen specific mab S2D2, a result which would suggest an idiotype − antiidiotype specific mechanism (6). By digestion of S-antigen with chymotrypsin and CNBr, it was possible to localize these epitopes in the N-terminal 74 amino acids (aa) of the protein (7). For identification of epitopes recognized by mab, a micromethod for epitope mapping was used which allows identification of sequential epitopes by systematic synthesis of all overlapping peptides of the N-terminal 74 aa on polyethylene rods, followed by immunoassays of all peptides with mab.

By this method, specific binding of mab S2D2 was reproducibly localized on peptides 40 to 44 (Fig. 1a), which correspond in the aa sequence to the residues 40 to 50. Specific mab binding was verified by dot blot, ELISA (Fig. 1b) and competition ELISA (Fig. 1c) using the corresponding synthetic peptide (S2) which was compared with peptides known to be pathogenic, i.e. K (S3, S4) and M regions. The epitope fine structure was studied with the aid of an amino acid replacement experiment (Fig. 1d). Amino acid residues P×DGV×L×D were identified as relevant for the binding of mab S2D2.

Conclusions: 1. Till now no mab reacting with the N-terminus and inhibiting EAU has been described by other authors. 2. According to L. DONOSO et al. (9), the N-terminal region including peptide S2 does not induce uveoretinitis. 3. Pathogenic regions so far identified, K and M peptides, are not recognized by S2 D2. These facts open the possibility that the S2 D2 epitope represents a tolerogenic region or that mab S2 D2 is interacting with pathogenic regions in a non identified manner. The determination of three-dimensional structure after crystallization of retinal S-antigen would help to understand the interaction of mab S2 D2 with S-antigen and its inhibitory effect on S-antigen induced EAU.

References

1. WACKER, W. B., DONOSO, L. A., KALSOW, C. M., YANKEELOW, J. A. Jr, ORGANISCIAK, D. T. (1977): J. Immunol. **119**, 1949
2. WILDEN, U., HALL, S. W., KÜHN, H. (1986): Proc. Natl. Acad. Sci. USA **83**, 1174
3. YAMAKI, K., TAKAHASHI, Y., SAKURAGI, S. MATSUBARA, K. (1987): Biochem. Biophys. Res. Commun. **142**, 904
4. MIRSHAHI, M., BOUCHEIX, C., COLLENOT, G., THILLAYE, B., FAURE, J. P. (1985): Invest. Ophthalmol. Vis. Sci. **26**, 1015
5. DE KOZAK, Y., MIRSHAHI, M., BOUCHEIX, C., FAURE, J. P. (1985): Eur. J. Immunol. **15**, 1107
6. DE KOZAK, Y., MIRSHAHI, M., BOUCHEIX, C., FAURE, J. P. (1987): Eur. J. Immunol. **17**, 541
7. MIRSHAHI, M., STIEMER, R., BERTRAND, O., LU HE, DE KOZAK, Y., FAURE, J. P. (1987): 29th Meet. Assoc. Eye Research, Louvain, Belgium
8. GEYSEN, H. M., RODDA, S. J., MASON, T. J., TRIBBICK, G., SCHOOFS, P. G. (1987): J. Immunol. Methods **102**, 259
9. DONOSO, L. A., MERRYMAN, C. F., SERY, T. W., SHINOHARA, T., DIETZSCHOLD, B., SMITH, A., KALSOW, C. M. (1987): Curr. Eye Res. **6**, 1151

Anti-Peptide Antibodies to Three CDR Sequences of Human Monoclonal Anti-DNA Autoantibodies

B. D. Stollar, A. Pucetti, and M. P. Madaio

Department of Biochemistry, Tufts University Health Science Campus, Boston, Massachusetts and the Department of Medicine, New England Medical Center Hospital, Boston, MA 02111, USA

Proteins 18/2 and 21/28 are monoclonal human IgM anti-DNA antibodies produced by hybridomas derived from an SLE patient. Antibody 18/2 bears an idiotype, 16/6, that has recurred on several different anti-DNA monoclonal antibodies, and on immunoglobulins in both the serum and tissue lesions of SLE patients. Both its heavy and light chain variable regions have been sequenced. Antibody 21/28 does not carry the 16/6 idiotype, but the center of its heavy chain CDR 3 is identical to that in 18/2. Its VH gene is from a different family than that of 18/2, but both proteins have similar amino acid sequences in and adjacent to the heavy chain CDR 1. To prepare serological reagents that could detect recurrence of related primary structures in other immunoglobulins, we have synthesized three peptides with sequences corresponding to the light chain CDR 3 of antibody 18/2 and to the heavy chain CDR 1 and CDR 3 of antibody 21/28. Rabbits were immunized with peptide-KLH conjugates of each of the peptides. Each antiserum reacted specifically with the immunizing peptide in direct and competitive ELISA, and with homologous intact IgM on dot blots. Anti-18/2 L-chain CDR 3 reacted with the 18/2 light chain on a Western blot, and detected no crossreacting molecules in a dot-blotted panel of 10 other human IgM immunoglobulins. Anti-21/28 H-CDR 3 reacted with both 21/28 and 18/2 proteins, which share sequence identity in this region, but it had the unpredicted property of reacting only with intact protein and not with heavy chain on a Western blot. A monoclonal murine antibody to the same peptide had the same property. The peptide is recognized in a conformation that occurs in native structure, but not in protein exposed to heat, SDS and mercaptoethanol. The third serum reacted with heavy chain on a Western blot, and cross-reacted with the heavy chain of 18/2, which has a similar sequence in this region even though it is encoded by a VH gene of a different family. The three anti-peptide sera are being tested as reagents for detection of recurrent primary structures.

Immunological Characterization of IgM Class Autoantibodies Against Sm-Antigenic B′/B and D Polypeptides of U Small Nuclear Ribonucleoproteins (snRNPs)

Y. Takeda, G. S. Wang, and G. C. Sharp

University of Missouri, Columbia, MO 65212, USA

IgG anti-Sm autoantibodies are known to react with epitope(s) shared by B′/B and D polypeptides of U snRNPs. With respect to the reactivities of IgM antibodies, only a few studies have been done at the polypeptide level. In this study, we investigated more detailed characteristics of IgM antibodies against Sm-antigenic B'/B and D polypeptides by enzyme-linked immunosorbent assay (ELISA).

Among 136 sera positive for antibodies to U snRNPs, the ratio of IgM and IgG ELISA levels (M/G) of B'/B was higher than M/G of D (P < 0.05). Furthermore, sera with high M/G of B'/B showed low IgM D ELISA levels. These results indicate that there are some sera with IgM B'/B but neither IgM D nor IgG B'/B reactivies. From these results, it appeared that there might be IgM autoantibodies directed against epitope(s) in B'/B polypeptides that differ from the Sm-epitope(s) shared with the D polypeptide, and that these antibodies might infrequently switch to IgG antibodies. In order to confirm this hypothesis, we performed competitive ELISAs using B'/B and D polypeptides.

In IgM B'/B ELISAs with inhibition by the D polypeptide performed on 99 sera with significant IgM B'/B reactivities (>mean+5 SD of negative control sera), 53 sera showed less than 40% inhibition ([ELISA level without inhibition − level with inhibition]/level without inhibition), 21 showed between 40% and 60%, and 25 showed more than 60% inhibition. Furthermore, sera with less than 40% inhibition showed lower IgG B'/B ELISA levels than sera with more than 60% inhibition (P < 0.05).

It was possible that these IgM reactions with B'/B polypeptides not inhibited by the D polypeptide might be due to non-specific reactions. Therefore, to rule out this possibility, IgM B'/B competitive ELISAs with inhibition by B'/B polypeptides were performed on 37 sera which had low % inhibition by the D polypeptide. All 37 sera showed more than 60% inhibition, indicating that these IgM reactivities against B'/B were specific.

In order to compare the IgM and IgG reactivities against B'/B polypeptides, we performed IgG B'/B competitive ELISAs with inhibition by the D polypeptide on the 23 sera with the highest IgG B'/B ELISA levels. Among the 23 sera, none showed less than 40%, 7 showed 40%−60%, and 16 showed more than 60% inhibition. On the other hand, in IgM B'/B competitive ELISAs with inhibition by the D polypeptide on the 23 sera with the highest IgM B'/B ELISA levels, 12 sera showed less than 40%, 3 showed 40−60%, and 8 showed more than 60% inhibition. These results suggest that the IgG antibodies to the B'/B polypeptides were mainly directed to Sm-epitope(s) shared with the D polypeptide: however, among IgM-reacting sera, there were a significant number whose IgM antibodies were directed to epitope(s) not shared with the D polypeptide.

Ten sera had significant IgM reactivities against both B'/B and D polypeptides, but less than 40% inhibition by the D polypeptide in IgM B'/B ELISAs. Among them, 3 sera showed less than 40% inhibition in IgM D ELISAs with competition by B'/B, suggesting that IgM reactivities to the D polypeptide in these sera were not related to epitope(s) shared with the B'/B polypeptides. By immunoblotting or ELISA without competition, these sera cannot be distinguished from sera with IgM reactivity against epitope(s) shared by B'/B and D. In longitudinal studies over more than 5 years in 3 patients with IgM reactivities to

B'/B but not to D, high IgG B'/B ELISA levels were not seen at any time, even though IgM B'/B reactivities remained high during this follow-up period.

This study provides further evidence for the infrequent switch from IgM to IgG of autoantibodies which react with epitope(s) unique to B'/B. Furthermore, it is possible that IgM autoantibodies to epitope(s) unique to the D polypeptide might also be present.

Enzyme-Linked Immunosorbent Assay Using Isolated (U) Small Nuclear Ribonucleoprotein Polypeptides as Antigens

Y. Takeda[1], J. Chen [1], G. S. Wang[1], R. J. Wang[1], S. K. Anderson[1], I. Pettersson[2], S. Amaki[1], and G. C. Sharp[1]

[1]University of Missouri, Columbia, MO 65212, USA
[2]Karolinska Institute, Stockholm, Sweden

Antibodies to U1 ribonucleoprotein (RNP) in very high titers have a strong association with mixed connective tissue disease (MCTD), and anti-Sm antibodies have a high specificity for systemic lupus erythematosus (SLE). These autoantibodies have been known to react with U small nuclear RNPs (snRNPs), and anti-RNP antibodies immunoprecipitate U1 RNA, while anti-Sm antibodies immunoprecipitate U1, U2, U4, U5, and U6 RNAs. Recent immunoblotting studies have revealed that anti-RNP antibodies react with 68 K, A, and C polypeptides, and anti-Sm antibodies react with B'/B and D polypeptides. Since immunoblotting is basically a qualitative assay, it is not suitable to investigate quantitative reactivities of autoimmune sera to individual U snRNP polypeptides. Thus, we have developed a quantitative ELISA for IgG and IgM antibodies using isolated 68 K, A, B'/B and D polypeptides as antigens. These polypeptide antigens for ELISA were eluted from gel after SDS-polyacrylamide electrophoreses of U1 snRNP affinity-purified from rabbit thymus extract. Purity and stability of these polypeptide antigens were confirmed by re-electrophoresis of each eluted polypeptide.

ELISA results using each U snRNP polypeptide were positively correlated with immunoblotting results. We performed the ELISA using isolated U snRNP polypeptides on sera from 59 anti-RNP-positive patients. Among the 59 patients, 33 had active MCTD, 5 had inactive MCTD, 12 had active SLE, and 9 had undifferentiated connective tissue disease (UCTD). In the 68 K polypeptide ELISA, patients with active MCTD showed significantly higher reactivity than patients with other diseases. On the other hand, in the A polypeptide ELISA, active MCTD and SLE patients did not show any difference in their reactivity. Since the typical serologic feature of MCTD is a high titer by passive hemagglutination of antibodies to extractable nuclear antigen (ENA-PHA), we compared the results of ENA-PHA titers and 68 K polypeptide ELISA levels. Although the anti-68 K ELISA levels correlated in general with ENA-PHA titers, there were some exceptions in which high ENA-PHA titers were associated with low anti-68 K ELISA levels. This discrepancy might be due to the presence in ENA of antigens other than the 68 K polypeptide. In the B'/B and D polypeptide ELISAs, patients with SLE showed higher reactivities than patients with other diseases.

In a comparison of clinical manifestation and U snRNP polypeptide ELISA results, patients with myositis and esophageal hypomotility showed significantly higher 68 K reactivity. Patients with renal disorder and patients without Raynaud's phenomenon showed higher B'/B and D polypeptide reactivities.

Longitudinal observations performed on 6 patients with MCTD revealed that IgG 68 K reactivity was related to disease activity.

We also utilized this ELISA for screening and characterization of human monoclonal antibodies to U snRNPs. An IgM class antibody-producing human lymphocyte cell line, designated Su-2E4, was isolated after Epstein-Barr virus transformation of lymphocytes from a patient with MCTD. In ELISAs using U snRNP polypeptides, Su-2E4 showed a high level of reactivity only in the case of the IgM 68 K polypeptide ELISA. This reactivity was inhibited by 50% when Su-2E4 was incubated with the 68 K polypeptide before being placed in antigen-coated wells, confirming the specificity of Su-2E4. To investigate the epitope relationship between Su-2E4 and a murine anti-68 K monoclonal antibody, 2.73, we preincubated 2.73 with the 68 K polypeptide-coated well before adding Su-2E4. The binding of su-2E4 to the 68 K polypeptide was inhibited by 64% by preincubation of the antigen with 2.73, suggesting that these two monoclonal antibodies are directed to closely related epitopes.

These results suggest that this specific ELISA using isolated U snRNP polypeptides is useful for the quantitative analysis of autoantibodies against these polypeptides. Using this method, we obtained quantitative confirmation of the relationship between IgG 68 K polypeptide reactivity and MCTD, and between IgG B'/B and D reactivities and SLE. Furthermore, this ELISA was useful for screening of monoclonal antibodies to U snRNPs, and facilitated quantitative competitive assays.

Analysis of U 1 Ribonucleoprotein (RNP) 68 K Polypeptide (p68 K) Epitopes by Enzyme-Linked Immunosorbent Assay (ELISA) with Fusion Proteins (FPs)

Y. Takeda[1], Y. Zhou[1], G. S. Wang[1], R. J. Wang[1], G. C. Sharp[1], I. Pettersson[2]

[1]University of Missouri, Columbia, MO 65212, USA
[2]Karolinska Institute, Stockholm, Sweden

Recent reports have shown a strong correlation between high levels of circulating autoantibodies to the U 1 RNP p68K and mixed connective tissue disease (MCTD), and murine and human monoclonal antibodies to p68K have been reported. Mechanisms of initiation and perpetuation of this autoimmune response, however, are not yet clear. Epitope mapping may be an approach to help elucidate those mechanisms. Thus, in order to analyze epitopes in the p68K, we performed an ELISA using as antigens fusion proteins encoded from fragments of cDNA for the p68K. The cDNA fragments were created by digestion with various restriction enzymes. Fusion proteins used in this study were FP 1 (amino acids 240−437), FP 2 (240−372), FP 3 (373−437), FP 5 (240−311), and FP 6 (272−372). For ELISA, we solubilized these fusion proteins by serial extraction using 1 M and 7 M urea. Sera with ELISA reactivities to protein expressed from vector pEX2 were excluded. We performed an IgG ELISA on 99 sera with IgG ELISA reactivity to p68K isolated after gel electrophoresis, and an IgM ELISA on 53 sera with IgM p68K reactivity.

FP 1 ELISA levels were correlated with p68K ELISA levels in the case of both IgG ($r = 0.83$, $P < 0.01$) and IgM ($r = 0.85$, $P < 0.01$), suggesting that anti-p68K autoantibodies are mainly directed to this region of the p68K.

We compared IgG and IgM ELISA reactivities against FP 2 and FP 3, which are 2 different fractions of FP 1 (FP 2 the N-terminal side and FP 3 the C-terminal side). In the case of both IgG and IgM, significant reactivities ($>$ mean $+ 5$ SD of negative control sera) were seen more frequently with FP 2 (92/99, IgG; 40/53, IgM) than with FP 3 (6/99, IgG; 11/53, IgM) ($P < 0.01$). Interestingly, both murine (2.73) and human (SU-2E4) monoclonal antibodies to p68K showed FP 3 reactivity. With respect to FP 3 reactivity, IgM was more frequent than IgG ($P < 0.01$), and among 11 sera with IgM FP 3 reactivity, only 1 showed an IgG FP 3 reaction. We performed competitive FP 2 and FP 3 ELISAs using isolated whole p68K as inhibiting antigen (performed on 7 sera for IgG FP 2, 4 for IgM FP 2, 4 for IgG FP 3, and 2 for IgM FP 3). These competitive ELISAs showed more than 50% inhibition, suggesting that these reactivities were specific for p68K, and that epitopes in FP 2 and FP 3 were similar to those in intact p68K.

In order to investigate serum reactivities to the FP 2 region in more detail, we did ELISAs using FP 5 and FP 6 which are smaller segments of FP 2. The frequency of sera with significant FP 5 reactivity was less (12/99, IgG; 11/53, IgM) than FP 2. On the other hand, FP 2 and FP 6 reactivities showed a positive correlation (r = 0.86, P > 0.01, IgG; r = 0.89, P > 0.01, IgM), indicating that the predominant epitopes for autoimmune sera were present in FP 6, but not in FP 5. In addition, because FP 5 contains a region of reported homology with retroviral p30^{gag} antigen, our results imply that cross-reactivities with the viral antigen might not be the primary mechanism of anti-p68K autoantibody production.

These results suggest that the main epitopes for serum IgG and IgM autoantibodies to p68K are located in the region of amino acids 312 – 372, whereas monoclonal antibodies are directed to the region of amino acids 373 – 437. Furthermore, autoantibodies to epitopes in the region of amino acids 373 – 437 appear to switch infrequently from IgM to IgG.

Contributions of Molecular and Cell Biology to Understanding of the B-Cell Response in Systemic Autoimmunity

E. M. Tan

W. M. Keck Autoimmune Disease, Research Institute of Scripps Clinic, La Jolla, CA 92037, USA

Systemic autoimmunity in diseases such as systemic lupus erythematosus, SJÖGRENs syndrome, scleroderma and dermato/polymyositis all have a very characteristic B-cell response which has two features: specificity and polyclonality. Specificity is demonstrated by the presence of antibodies such as anti-Sm and anti-native DNA which are almost exclusively seen in patients with lupus and antibodies to Scl-70 and centromere proteins which are almost exclusively seen in scleroderma. Polyclonality is manifested by the presence of antibodies reactive with at least ten different antigens in the case of lupus and against several epitopes on individual antigens. Similarly, autoantibodies in scleroderma are directed to at least seven different antigens, with several epitopes demonstrated on at least one of these, the centromere B protein.

What is immunologically defined as the Sm antigen has been shown to consist of several proteins B, B′, D and E (28, 29, 16 and 13 kD) which are components of U 1, U 2, U 4, U 5 and U 6 small nuclear ribonucleoprotein (snRNP) particles. These particles contain a family of "uridine-rich" nuclear RNAs. Similarly, the SS-B/La antigen has also been shown to be a subcellular particle composed of a 48 kD phosphoprotein frequently complexed with nascent RNA pol III transcripts, which include precursor tRNAs, 5 S RNA and 7 S RNA. These and other information elucidating the nature of intracellular antigens argue strongly for the hypothesis that the autoimmune response is antigen driven and that the *in vivo* antigen is a subcellular particle. These subcellular particles are different in different disease states so that in lupus, one of the forms of subcellular particles is snRNP while in SJÖGRENs syndrome the particles are those involved in pol III transcription. The antigen-driven hypothesis could also explain the polyclonality of the autoimmune response, since there are many component parts to subcellular particles including proteins and nucleic acids. In the immune response in SJÖRGRENs syndrome, the simultaneous occurrence of antibodies to SS-A/Ro and SS-B/La, a feature frequently observed in this disease, is explained by the probable complexing of the SS-A and SS-B particles *in vivo* and presented to the immune system as such, so that antibody to SS-B is almost always coupled with the co-expression of antibody to SS-A.

Many investigators have observed that autoantibodies inhibit the function of their cognate antigens. These include inhibition of precursor mRNA splicing by antibodies to Sm and U 1-RNP, inhibition of aminoacylation of tRNA by autoantibodies to tRNA synthetases, inhibition of 28 S and 18 S RNA synthesis by autoantibody to RNA polymerase 1 and inhibition of *in vitro* and *in vivo* DNA replication by antibody to proliferating cell nuclear antigen (PCNA) or auxiliary protein of DNA polymerase δ. The meaning of these observations was clarified in several studies showing that autoantibodies were recognizing unique sites on the antigens whereas experimentally-induced monoclonal antibodies which were not inhibitory were recognizing different epitopes. This type of information associating recognition of unique epitopes and inhibition of function of the antigen has been shown for autoantibodies to PCNA, threonyl-tRNA synthetase and the pyruvate dehydrogenase antigen related to primary biliary cirrhosis.

Base on these considerations, the autoimmune response is very likely to be antigen-driven and the immunogen *in vivo* appears to be a subcellular particle. The autoimmune response is directed at various components of the subcellular particles, but the active or catalytic sites of these particles are often the targets of the B-cell response.

Immunospecificity and Clinical Association of Autoantibodies in Sera Precipitating U1 and U2 Small Nuclear RNAs

T. Tojo, T. Ogasawara, Y. Okano, T. Mimori, and M. Homma

Keio University School of Medicine, Tokyo, Japan

Autoantibodies to U small nuclear ribonucleoproteins (UsnRNP) are known to have close clinical associations in certain rheumatic diseases. Antigenic epitopes of anti-U2RNP antibody have been shown to be present in A′ (31 kD) or B″ (28.5 kD) polypeptides of U2 snRNP molecule from HeLa cells. However due to the cross reactive epitopes present both in the B″ of U2 RNP and the A (33 kD) peptides U1 RNP, sera with anti-U2 RNP also immunoprecipitate U1 RNA. Because of this crossreactivity and the limited number of patients with the sera, the exact clinical implication of the antibodies still remains unsatisfactory.

To get a better understanding of immunospecificities and clinical associations of the antibodies in sera that immunoprecipitate both U1 and U2 snRNAs, patients with systemic rheumatic diseases were investigated. Sera from these patients were screened for UsnRNAs by immunoprecipitation method using ^{32}p-labelled HeLa cell extracts. We found 10 sera that precipitated only U1 and U2 RNAs but not U4, U5 and U6. Immunospecificities of these sera could not be differentiated from those containing only anti-U1 RNP antibodies by conventional double immunodiffusion or passive hemagglutination tests. By immunoblotting analysis using substrates enriched for either U1 or U2 RNP, all ten sera were shown to react with both B″ and A peptides indicating the presence of common antibodies to U1/U2 RNP in these sera. Nine sera were also shown to react with 68 k peptides of U1 RNP indicating the presence of antibodies to U1 RNP. This reactivity to 68 k peptides could be confirmed by enzyme-linked immunosorbent assay using isolated peptides as the antigen.

The clinical characteristics of these patients were compaired with those of patients having anti-U1 RNP or anti-U1 U2 U4-6 RNP (Sm) antibodies. Incidence of sclerotic skin changes confined to fingers or forearms and mild myopathy with slightly increased serum levels of creatinine phosphokinase was significantly higher than that in both groups of patients with anti-U1 RNP or anti-U1 U2 U4-6 RNP (Sm) antibodies.

The results confirmed the previously reported immunospecificity of anti-U2 RNP antibody and indicate that patients with anti-U1/U2 RNP antibodies may be classified into an unique clinical subset in heterogeneous groups of patients with overlapping features including those with mixed connective tissue disease.

Anti-Jo-1 Antibodies are Directed at an Evolutionarily-Conserved, Conformational Site on Human Histidyl-tRNA Synthetase

K. Waite, F. W. Miller, and P. H. Plotz, N. I. H.

Arthritis and Rheumatism Branch, Clinical Center 9N244, National Institutes of Health, Bethesda, MD 20892, USA

Anti-Jo-1 antibodies (AJoA) directed against the cellular enzyme histidyl-tRNA synthetase (HRS) are found in approximately 25% of patients with idiopathic myositis. They occur in a distinct subset of patients whose inflammatory muscle disease is often accompanied by interstitial lung disease, arthritis, and Raynaud's phenomenon. Less commonly, patients in this clinical group have an autoantibody to a different aminoacyl-tRNA synthetase. The autoantibodies target proteins which are functionally but not antigenically related.

In previous studies, we have shown that all antisera which bind to histidyl-tRNA synthetase by western blotting or ELISA inhibit its enzymatic activity, and that all antisera appear to recognize the same proteolytic fragments of the polypeptide.

In order to identify any linear epitopes recognized by AJoA, all possible overlapping hexapeptides corresponding to the 508 amino acid sequence of human HRS, as determined by Tsui and Siminovich, were synthesized. These hexapeptides were tested in an ELISA assay with IgG isolated from the sera of myositis patients positive for AJoA, myositis patients negative for AJoA, and normal volunteers. In addition, antibodies raised in rabbits against two decapeptides of human HRS which were predicted to be antigenic were assessed for reactivity against the appropriate solid phase peptides.

As expected, the rabbit anti-peptide Abs reacted strongly with the correct hexapeptides corresponding to the immunogen. The Abs raised against peptide A (residues 18–27) bound to hexapeptides starting with residues 18 through 24, whereas the pre-immune sera from the same rabbit showed no reactivity to these peptides. Thus, a minimum of four amino acid residues could be recognized by Abs in this system. Similarly, Abs against peptide B (residues 436–445) bound to hexapeptides starting with residue 435 through 441. Additional reactivity was observed, however. The hexapeptides showing this additional reactivity posses no sequence homology to the immunizing decamer and may, therefore, have been recognized by other antibodies raised in response to the KLH and Freund's adjuvant used for immunization.

Each of four AJoA positive sera tested showed a similar pattern of reactivity across the entire sequence of HRS. The same pattern of reactivity was observed, however, when the peptides were tested with the IgG from the sera of normal controls (N-5) and AJoA-negative myositis patients (N-2), and from the AJoA-negative serum drawn from a patient who subsequently became AJoA positive. No hexapeptides reacted solely with AJoA positive sera, indicating that no linear epitopes of this molecule are recognized by AJoA.

In order to characterize further the target or the antibodies, we examined the ability of AJoA to inhibit the function of HRS from various species. Other studies had shown that the bovine as well as human but not the *E. coli* enzyme are bound and inhibited by AJoA. AJoA inhibited the aminoacylation of histidine to its respective tRNA in human, anole, frog, and fish cytoplasmic extracts by 90.0%, 89.1%, 82.5%, and 52.2% respectively. No inhibition of HRS enzyme activity was observed for yeast, euglena, amoeba, algae, or *E. coli* extracts.

These data suggest that these autoantibodies recognize a conformational, not a linear, epitope of HRS, critical to enzyme function, conserved throughout the animal kingdom, but not present in the other four kingdoms. The ability of AJoA to inhibit HRS activity through phylogeny suggests that the autoantibodies recognize a relatively conserved region of the antigen. The preferential inhibition of human HRS and the decreasing inhibition as phylogenetic distance from man increases suggest that the human enzyme may have a critical role in this antibody response.

Molecular Considerations of Primary Biliary Cirrhosis: Definition of Dihydrolipoamide Acetyltransferase and Identification of Immunoreactive Sites

J. Van de Water, P. Leung, A. Ansari, R. L. Coppel, and M. E. Gershwin

Div. Rheumatology-Clinical Immunology, University of California, Davis, California; Dept. Pathology, Emory University, Atlanta, GA; Hall Institute, Melbourne, Australia

Autoantibodies to mitochondrial antigens are characteristic of primary biliary cirrhosis, but the precise antigenic determinants recognized by these antibodies have not ben defined. We have identified and sequenced both human and rat genes that code for a polypeptide recognized specifically by sera from patients with PBC but not by sera from patients with other forms of liver disease. This recombinant protein was identified as the 74 kD M2 mitochondrial inner membrane autoantigen, dihydrolipoamide acetyltransferase. We have identified a 603 bp fragment (pRMIT-603) which codes for a polypeptide containing all of the autoreactivity of the original clone. Based on hydrophobicity/hydrophilicity plots of the amino acid sequence of this polypeptide segment, several peptides were synthesized and tested for reactivity by an inhibition assay using sera from patients with PBC. One peptide, defined by the amino acids (AEIETDKATIGFEV-QEEGYL), obsorbed serum reactivity to the fusion protein of the original clone. This peptide contains the lipoic acid binding site KATIGF of the dihydrolipo-amide acetyltransferase found in the inner mitochondrial membrane. Of particular interest, inhibition of PDH activity was demonstrated after incubation with sera from patients with PBC but not from normal volunteers or patients with chronic active hepatitis (CAH). Such inhibition was abrogated by absorption of the PBC sera with pRMIT-603. Thus, it appears that for this autoantigen, the target of the autoantibodies corresponds to a functional site of the dihydrolipo-amide acetyltransferase. Dihydrolipoamide is a very well-conserved antigen and the identification of immunoreactive sites provides the opportunity to address the molecular basis of self-recognition and putative mechanisms of biliary duct destruction.

Association of Seropositive Rheumatoid Arthritis (RA) with the Third Hypervariable Region (HVR3) of the HLA-DR β1-Chain: Functional Implications for Antigen-Specific and Allogeneic T Cell Recognition

C. M. Weyand, J. J. Goronzy

Div. of Rheum., Dept. of Med., University of Heidelberg, FRG

The genetic predisposition to develop seropositive rheumatoid arthritis (RA) is inherited within two different alleles, HLA-DR 1 and HLA-DR 4. Sequence analysis and studies with T cell clones have demonstrated that the association for RA can be localized to the HLA-DR β1-chain. The genetic polymorphism of the HLA-DR β1-chain is clustered in three hypervariable regions which might correlate to different functional domains of the HLA-molecule on the cell surface. We have now used antigen-specific T cell clones generated from patients with RA and allogeneic T cell clones raised against cells of patients with RA to address the question which functional properties of the HLA-DR β1-chain are associated with RA. By the use of alloreactive T cell clones a cluster of T cell epitopes can be defined which are shared amongst the RA-associated haplotypes HLA-DR 1, Dw 4, Dw 13, Dw 14 and Dw 15. Sequence homologies between the HVR 3 of the RA-associated haplotypes allowed to map the crossreactive T cell epitopes to that functional region. However, the RA-associated T cell epitopes could not be strictly correlated to the primary amino acid sequence indicating that the disease-associated epitopes are conformational. As suggested by threedimensional models of the HLA-molecule, the HVR 3 might be involved in the interaction with the T cell receptor as well as the selected antigenic peptide. To investigate the functional role of RA-associated T cell epitopes, antigen-specific T cells were established in three antigenic systems: tetanus toxoid, Epstein-Barr virus and mycobacterial antigens. Series of antigen-specific T cell clones were generated from DR 1 $^+$ and DR 4 $^+$ RA patients. When these clones were tested for their proliferative response none of the clones was able to recognize antigen when presented by stimulator cells similar for the HVR 3 but distinct for the HVR 2 and HVR 1. In a next step polyclonal T cell lines from DR 1/DR 4 heterozygous RA patients were generated. These lines were either restricted to HLA-DR 1 or DR 4 and could not be maintained when crosstimulated with the alternative haplotype suggesting that antigen-specific HLA-DR 1 and DR 4 crossreactive T cells are not represented in the T cell repertoire. These data suggest that the shared conformational T cell epitopes associated with RA are encoded by a functional domain of the HLA-molecule which is not involved in selecting an "arthritogenic antigenic peptide".

The snRNP E Protein: Structure and Expression of a Human Autoimmune Antigen

E. D. Wieben, D. R. Stanford, M. Fautsch, C. Perry, J. Patton, K. Neiswanger, E. Holicky, A. Rohleder, R. Sparkes, I. Klisak, B. Knerer, and A. Chang-Miller

Department of Biochemistry and Molecular Biology, Mayo Foundation/Clinic, Rochester, MN 55905, USA

The snRNP E protein is both an snRNP core protein and a known autoimmune antigen. This 10 800 dalton basic protein is recognized by a subset of patient anti-Sm sera. A partial cDNA clone coding for the E protein was originally isolated from a size-selected cDNA library from HeLa cells. This cDNA clone has been used as a starting point for investigations of the primary stucture of the protein, the interaction of this protein with other components of snRNPs, and the structure and expression of the E protein multigene family.

A full-length cDNA clone isolated from a human teratoma cDNA library has been fully sequenced. The predicted amino acid sequence from this clone codes for a basic 92 amino acid polypeptide that contains regions of sequence similarity to at least one eukaryotic ribosomal protein. Comparison of the primary sequence of the E protein to that of the other Sm proteins does not reveal any extensive regions of sequence homology. However, the region of greatest homology to the snRNP B and D proteins is at the carboxyl terminus of the E protein. Site-directed monoclonal antibodies against the carboxyl terminus of the E protein have now been produced. These antibodies show some cross-reaction with other small RNA-binding proteins from HeLa cells. We are currently investigating the identify of these proteins.

Eight of 10 genomic clones for the human E protein have the structure expected for processed pseudogenes. One clone contains an E protein coding sequence that spans 9 kb and is interrupted by four introns. The 5′ flanking region of this clone contains several sequence similarities to promoter elements found invertebrate ribosomal protein genes and snRNA genes. Analysis of the promoter region from this E gene by transfection of kidney 293 cells with CAT fusion constructs suggests that the regions of sequence similarity to snRNA and ribosomal protein genes may have functional relevance.

The intron-containing gene for the E protein has been mapped to chromosome 1 by both hybridization to a panel of somatic cell hybrids and by in situ hybridization. The in situ hybridization results suggest that the gene is located in the region 1q2.5−q4.3. Thus, this gene is physically linked to a number of genes coding for U1 RNA.

A tenth genomic clone contains only the 3′ terminal 113 nts of the E protein cDNA sequence. The E protein homologous sequence is flanked on the 3′ terminus by a poly(A) tract of 16 nts and on the 5′ end by a variant gene for another component of the RNA processing machinery, U6 snRNA. The coding region of the U6 gene is 90% homologous to a previously characterized human U6 gene, but lacks any homology to the 5′ flanking elements previously shown to be required for efficient U6 transcription. However, the variant U6 gene is efficiently transcribed by RNA polymerase III in a HeLa cell S100 extract, and can compete with cloned tRNA genes for transcription factors. Additional interest in this unusual genomic clone is generated by the finding that the U6-E protein sequences are located in the seventh intron of the human guanine nucleotide binding protein $G_i3\alpha$.

Studies of the interaction of the E protein with other components of snRNPs suggest that the E protein does not directly bind to snRNAs. Studies of the interaction of the E protein with other cloned snRNP proteins are in progress.

Autoantibodies to Nonhistone Chromosomal Proteins HMG-1 and HMG-2 in Subsets of Juvenile Chronic Arthritis (JCA)

B. Wittemann[1], F. A. Bautz[1], H. Michels[2], and H. Truckenbrodt[2]

[1] Institute of Molekular Genetiks, University of Heidelberg, Im Neuenheimer Feld 230, 6900 Heidelberg, FRG
[2] Rheumatic Children Hospital Garmisch-Partenkirchen, Gehfeldstraße 24, 8100 Garmisch-Partenkirchen, FRG

Antihistone antibodies (AHAs) in sera of patients suffering from juvenile chronic arthritis (JCA) have been reported recently by several investigators [1, 2].

In our study of 100 patients with JCA admitted to the Rheumatic Children's Hospital in Garmisch-Partenkirchen we observed, in addition to antibodies against various histones, autoantibodies against the nucleosomal proteins HMG-1 and HMG-2. All sera tested were ANA positive by indirect immunofluorescence on HEp-2 cells and negative when tested against double stranded DNA by an indirect solid phase ELISA (Progen GmbH, Heidelberg). In the analysis reported here we submitted purified HMG-1 and HMG-2 from calf-thymus [3] to PAGE and subsequent western blots. The results presented in the table give a correlation between clinical diagnosis and the presence of autoantibodies to nucleosomal proteins HMG-1 and HMG-2 in JCA patients.

Table 1

Clinical diagnosis	tested (no)	positive (no)	HMG-1 only	HMG-2 only	HMG-1 + HMG-2
Polyarthritis	14 (2*)	4 (2*)	1	0	3
Oligoarthritis	86 (13*)	37 (3*)	10	7	20

* JCA with uveitis.

Grouping the sera tested according to the clinical diagnosis (Table 1) reveals a correlation between detectable amounts of antibodies to the chromosomal proteins HMG-1 and HMG-2 and subsets of JCA. JCA patients with polyarthritis react to 28%, whereas patients with oligoarthritis show a higher incident of 43% binding to the high mobility group proteins 1 and 2.

References

1. OSTENSEN, M. et al. (1989): Identification of antihistone antibodies in subsets of juvenile chronic arthritis. Annals of the Rheumatic diseases **48**, 114–117
2. PAULS, J.D., FRITZLER, M.J. (1989): Juvenile Rheumatoid Arthritis antibodies bind Histones H1 and H5. Arth. & Rheum. 32, No 1
3. BUSTIN, M. et al. (1982): Autoantibodies to Nucleosomal Proteins: Antibodies to HMG-17 in Autoimmunie Diseases. Science **215**, 1245–1247

A Human T Cell Clone Recognizing Small Nuclear Ribonucleoproteins (UsnRNP)

G. Wolff-Vorbeck[1], M. Schlesier[1], W. Hackl[2], R. Lührmann[2], and H.H. Peter[1]

[1] Abt. Rheumatologie und klinische Immunologie, Medizinische Universitätsklinik, Freiburg, FRG
[2] Institut für Molekularbiologie und Tumorforschung, Philipps Universität, Marburg, FRG

Autoantibodies to U1 snRNP are frequently found in patients with mixed connective tissue disease (MCTD) and systemic lupus erythematosus (SLE). So far it is not known, whether this autoantibody production is T cell-dependent.

From peripheral blood of a healthy donor we established a CD3$^+$ T cell line, composed of both CD4$^+$ and CD8$^+$ cells, which recognizes unfractionated UsnRNP. By inhibition studies with monoclonal antibodies and testing of a panel of HLA typed individuals, the cell line was shown to be HLA-DR4 restricted. The cell line does not recognize control antigens such as PPD, collagen type II, proteoglycan or mycobacterial 65 kD heat shock protein. From this T cell line an UsnRNP-specific CD4$^+$ T cell clone has been derived; its fine specificity is under investigation using fractionated UsnRNP proteins. In addition, the autoantigenspecific helper activity of the T cell clone for immunoglobulin production by autologous B cells will be studied in vitro.

Epitope Progression in Autoantibody Production Suggested by Epitope Mappings of SS-B/La and U 2snRNP B″ Protein

K. Yamamoto[1], H. Kohsaka[1], H. Miura[1], H. Fujii[1], Y. Misaki[1], N. Miyasaka[2], K. Nishioka[2], and T. Miyamoto[1]

[1] Department of Medicine and Physical Therapy, Faculty of Medicine, University of Tokyo, Japan
[2] Institute of Rheumatology, Tokyo Women's Medical College, Tokyo, Japan

In order to understand the mechanisms of autoantibody productions in autoimmune patients, we cloned cDNAs encoding the SS-B/La and the U2 snRNP B″ proteins. The initial cloning was performed with λgt11 cDNA libraries from human fibroblasts and autoimmune patients' sera. The isolated clones were characterized with the purified antibodies against the fusion proteins produced by the cDNAs in *E. coli*. The clones identified to encode the SS-B/La or U2snRNP B″ protein were then used as probes for obtaining full length cDNAs from Okayama-Berg cDNA libraries. A clone termed FS4 was found to encode the entire coding region of the U2snRNP B″ protein. A clone called FSB was also determined to contain the whole coding region of the SS-B/La protein. To obtain large amount of the antigen molecules in *E. coli*, we have subcloned these FS4 and FSB into another expression vector pEX. Positive clones producing fusion proteins with cro-β-galactosidase were selected with patients' sera.

Enzyme linked immunosorbent assay (ELISA) was established with these fusion proteins. FS4EX and FSBEX. In the case of the SS-B/La protein, it was found that there is a good correlation between the reactivities of patients sera to FSBEX and the conventionally determined specificities of the sera. However, for the U2snRNP B″ protein, about 50% of anti-RNP positive sera were found to react with FS4EX, which is rather high frequency compared to the previous reports.

For epitope mapping, the pEX plasmids containing the cDNAs were enzymatically manipulated to produce deletion mutants. The resultant several deletion mutants were examined for the reactivities with many patients' sera. It was found that the U2snRNP B″ protein contains two main epitopes closely located in the C terminus. The SS-B/La protein was also shown to possess two major epitopes located in the N terminal and C terminal region respectively. Every patients' sera possessing the reactivities to these proteins recognized the major epitope(s). However, there were some patients' sera which additionally recognized other epitopes on the molecules. So far, these patients seemed to be rather advanced in the clinical courses. In addition, in the case of the U2snRNP B″ protein, the main epitopes were found to be cross-reactive to the U1snRNP A protein. Thus, it is possible that the initial reactivity to the B″ protein is in the main epitopes by the cross-reactive antibodies to the U1snRNP A protein. Thereafter, the whole molecule could become immunogenic to the host and the other parts of the protein would then be recognized. The reacting pattern by patients' sera to the SS-B/La protein also suggests this possibility. From these studies, it is postulated that there exist epitope progression phenomena in the autoantibody production.

Association of Autoantigenic Epitope and Catalytic Site on Poly (ADP-Ribose) Polymerase

H. Yamanaka[1], E. H. Willis[2], and D. A. Carson[2]

[1] Institute of Rheumatology, Tokyo Women's Medical College, NS bldg., 2-4-1 Nishi-shinjuku, Shinjuku-ku, Tokyo 163, Japan
[2] Research Institute of Scripps Clinic, 10666 North Torrey Pines Road, La Jolla, CA 92037, USA

Poly(ADP-ribose) polymerase is an eukaryotic DNA-binding enzyme, and transfers the ADP-ribose moiety of NAD to nuclear proteins. This nuclear enzyme is strongly activated by DNA with single- or double stand breaks, and has been postulated to play important roles on DNA repair and DNA replication. We have identified human autoantibodies to poly(ADP-ribose) polymerase in the sera of seven rheumatic patients. No other autoantibodies were detected in these patients sera. The specificity of the autoantibodies to poly(ADP-ribose) polymerase was established by a) immunoprecipitation and b) immunoprecipitation of enzyme activity of poly(ADP-ribose) polymerase.

Nuclear proteins are common targets of autoimmune responses in patients with systemic rheumatic diseases. However, it is still unclear how abnormal immune regulation leads to the repeated production of autoantibodies against such a highly selected group of self-components. Although the clinical significance of autoantibodies to poly(ADP-ribose) polymerase have not been established, the occurrence of highly specific autoantibodies to this well characterized nuclear enzyme is an excellent opportunity to investigate the pathogenesis of the autoantibody production. Since the entire structure of poly(ADP-ribose) polymerase is known, and cDNA of this protein is isolated, we could examine the epitope specificity of the human autoantibodies, and their effects on the biological functions of this nuclear enzyme.

Previous experiments have shown that poly(ADP-ribose) polymerase has three distinctive functional domains, DNA-binding, automodification and NAD-binding domains, by enzymatic digestion of the protein. All sera with autoantibodies to poly(ADP-ribose) polymerase recognized the NAD-binding domain of the enzyme, as demonstrated by either immunoblotting or immunoprecipitation experiments of partially proteolyzed poly(ADP-ribose) polymerase. The autoantibodies also inhibited the catalytic activity of the purified calf enzyme, as measured by the transfer of ADP-ribose from [^{32}P]NAD to either histones or to poly(ADP-ribose) polymerase itself.

Because comparative structural analyses have shown that the active sites of enzymes are often conserved during evolution, we tested the ability of the autoantibodies to react with poly(ADP-ribose) polymerase from lower eukaryotes. The human autoantibodies react with poly(ADP-ribose) polymerase in cellular extract from mammalian, avian, amphibian, arthropod, and protozoan cells, and also inhibit the catalytic activity of the various enzymes. Furthermore, the analysis of the cDNA of poly(ADP-ribose) polymerase revealed that an autoantigenic fragment of this protein is reminiscent of other NAD-utilizing dehydrogenases in the predicted secondary structure. These experiments indicate that the human autoantibodies to poly(ADP-ribose) polymerase recognize a distinctive group of evolutionarily conserved antigenic determinants that are closely related to the catalytic site of the enzyme. The results are consistent with the hypothesis that the epitope selectivity of human autoantibodies to poly(ADP-ribose) polymerase is influenced by cross-reactive antigens in the external environment.

Rheumatoid Arthritis is Associated with the Presence of Anti-Nuclear Antibodies to A 33 kD Protein (RA33) and Related Antigens

W. Hassfeld, G. Steiner, and J. S. Smolen

2nd Department of Medicine, University of Vienna, and 2nd Department of Medicine – Center for Rheumatic Diseases, Lainz Hospital, Vienna, Austria

Autoantibodies to nuclear antigens (ANA) represent hallmarks of several inflammatory rheumatic diseases. Particular ANA-subsets are characteristic for certain disorders, such as anti-Sm for systemic lupus erythematosus, anti-Scl70 for scleroderma, and anti-SSB for primary SJÖGREN's syndrome. In contrast to these "connective tissue diseases", rheumatoid arthritis (RA) has not been associated with antibodies to nuclear antigens, nor is there a pathogenomic autoantibody known for this disorder. In the present investigation we have analysed sera from patients with RA for the presence of antibodies to nuclear proteins. To this end, the immunoblot technique was employed using HeLa cell nuclear extracts as antigenic source. In 35% of sera from RA patients but in only 1 from 150 various controls a band corresponding to the molecular weight of 33 kD was found and the respective antigen termed RA 33. Further investigations revealed reactivity of RA sera with at least two additional nuclear antigens in the molecular weight range of 30 to 40 kD. These bands were commonly associated with RA 33. Antibodies to RA 33 and/or one or both of these additional antigens were observed in 31 of 50 sera tested (62%) but were not found in 40 control sera. The described antigens were resistant to digestion with RNase, DNase, freezethawing and heating to 56 °C and did not appear related to known nuclear antigens.

These data reveal that RA is related to the other connective tissue diseases by virtue of the presence of characteristic autoantibodies to nuclear proteins. Further studies will deal with the characterisation of the antigen(s) and their potential pathogenetic role.

Molecular Cloning and Identification of Retroviral Nucleic Acids Associated with Systemic Lupus Erythematosus

M. Herrmann, W. Leitmann, E.F. Krapf, and J.R. Kalden

Institute for Clinical Immunology, Dept. of Int. Med. III, University of Erlangen-Nürnberg, Erlangen, FRG

One characteristic of systemic lupus erythematosus (SLE), the induction of DNA antibodies, is probably triggered by foreign events. Recently we isolated high molecular weight plasma nucleic acids (PNA) of SLE patients with unusual features [1]. Molecular cloning and sequencing showed that one M 13 clone (E 6) of PNA had homology to the human immunodeficiency virus 1 (HIV 1) *pol-gag* overlap [2] (Fig. 1).

So we performed *in vitro* transfection of a human B cell line from a healthy donor (B 62) with these PNA. These experiments showed that PNA were able to induce alterations in B 62 cells similar to retroviralinfections. Northern blots demonstrated the induction of E 6 homologous mRNA in transfected cells (B 62/SLE). To characterize the mRNAs, a cDNA library was established from B 62/SLE cells and cloned into lambda gt 10. A single stranded E 6 DNA or an E 6 derived synthetic oligonucleotide was used to sceen these libraries. Two clones, lgt 10/3 and lgt 10/4, containing 8 and 9 kbp inserts, could be isolated from the library. The inserts were subcloned into pT 7 T3 18u and will be sequenced after

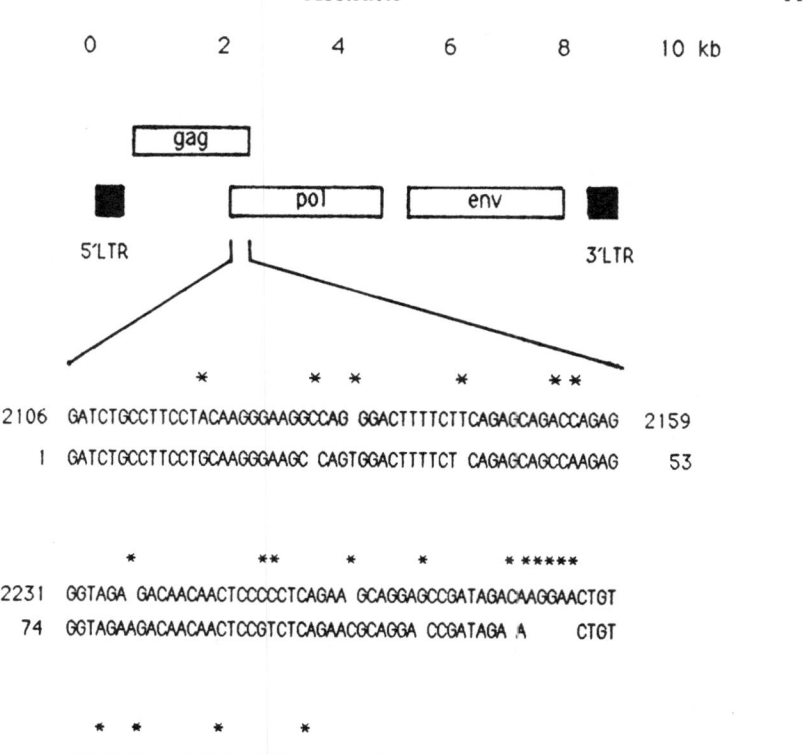

Fig. 1. The homology of E 6 (152–297) to the proviral genome of HIV 1 (2106–2309).
Mismatches are indicated by asterisks

nested deletions made with Exonuclease III and Nuclease S 1 from the single stranded templates induced by a helper phage.

Since it was not possible to detect integrated, nuclear DNA in the transfected cells by Southern blotting, possibly due to the low percentage of infected cells, we applied the polymerase chain reaction (PCR) technique for DNA amplification using oligonucleotide primers derived from the E 6 sequence. In both B 62/cells and 7 put of 30 B cell lines from 10 different SLE patients, amplification products of 150 to 500 bp were found; a similar pattern was observed in peripheral blood lymphycte (PBL) samples from AIDS patients, who served as positive controls, and PBL samples of an SLE patient, as well as one patient with clinical signs of rheumatoid arthritis. No DNA amplification products were found in samples of healthy individuals so far (n = 5); therefore, PCR proved to be useful for rapid detection of E 6 homologous DNA and supported the hypothesis of a retroviral participation in the pathogenesis of SLE.

References

1. KRAPF, F. E., HERRMANN, M., LEITMANN, W., KALDEN, J. R.: Clin. Exp. Immunol. (in press)
2. HERRMANN, M., LEITMANN, W., KRAPF, E. F., KALDEN, J. R.: J. Cell. Mol. Biol. (in press)

Molecular Features of an RNA Recognition Motif Family of Proteins

J. D. Keene

Department of Microbiology and Immunology, Duke University Medical Center, Durham, NC 27710, USA

A family of modular proteins has been recognized that can interact in a specific manner with RNA and in some cases with other molecules. These proteins contain a common primary sequence motif (RRM) of 80 amino acids that is part of the RNA binding domain. Several members of the family are autoantigenic in that they are components of small nuclear ribonucleoproteins of human cells. The autoreactive members of the family include the 70 K, A, La, Ro and B'' proteins.

The RRM family of proteins can be divided into two classes, those that contain a single copy of the RRM and those that contain two or more copies. Among the members of the family that are known to be autoimmune, the La, 60 K Ro and 70 K RNP proteins are within class I while the A and B'' proteins are within class II. Most members of the RRM family have some apparent role in RNA processing although some members have also been implicated in transcription (La, rho and Ro). It is possible that the entire family evolved from a common ancestral gene within a functional network involving RNA processing.

The sites of recognition of RNA by several members of the RRM family have been elucidated using a variety of methods including Northwestern blotting, immunoprecipitation of complexes and mobility shift assays. Together with nuclease protection and *in vitro* synthesis of specific deletion mutants of the RNAs, binding sites have been assigned. These approaches have recently yielded definitive assignments with the availability of recombinant vectors expressing the La, Ro, 70 K, A and B'' proteins.

The RNA recognition motif is a candidate region for cross-reactivity among the autoantigenic members of the family. However, since several members of the family do not appear to react with autoimmune sera and because many autoantigenic proteins do not contain an RRM, this possibility appears remote. One epitope identified by VAN VENROOIJ and coworkers resides within the RRM of the A protein and also reacts with the B″ protein. However, these antibodies do not seem to recognize other members of the RRM family. It cannot be ruled out at this time whether antibodies that cross-react within RRM are present at early stages in the development of autoimmune disease and then disappear at later times.

The autoantigenic members of the RRM family of proteins appear to be common to most tissues and conserved among metazoans. They probably constitute important housekeeping functions that are required for constitutive RNA metabolic processes. Recently, other members of the family have become evident that may interact with or modify the normal functioning of the constitutive RNA processing functions. For example, the Drosophila proteins involved in sex determination, and perhaps, some viral proteins may influence the pattern of splice site selection through interactions with components of the small nuclear RNPs, in particular, the 70 K protein of U1 snRNPs. Some of these proteins include the transformer, transformer-2, and sex-lethal proteins, as well as, gag gene products of retroviruses. Transformer-2 and sex-lethal proteins contain RRM sequences and presumably interact directly with RNA (see figure), while transformer and gag contain arginine-rich (RD/RS/RE) sequences similar to those present in the carboxyl region of 70 K, but lack an RRM. The sequence relationships and the proposed trans-acting functions exhibited by these proteins in the determination of splice site selection will be discussed. Below is a diagramatic representation of

RRM Family Proteins

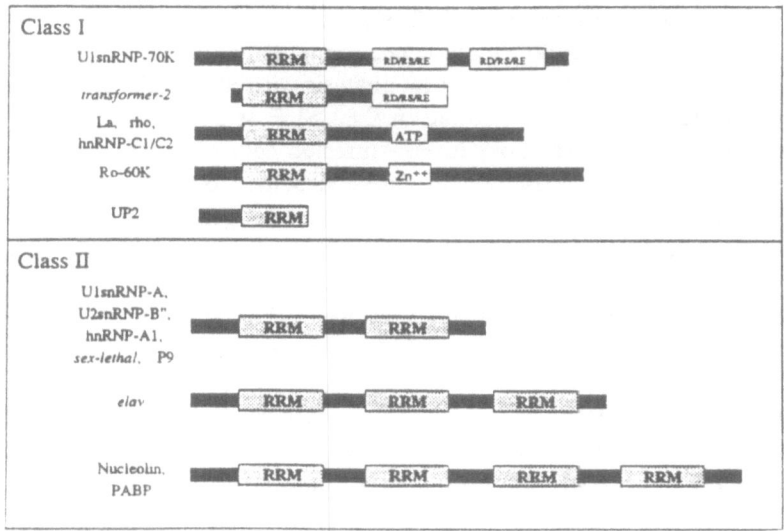

some of the members of this family of proteins and the distinction of classes I and II. Exciting developments in this field are expected to emerge from study of the RNA binding properties of the potentially multivalent members of class II of this RRM family proteins. Recent findings will be presented that the amino terminal RRM of the class II snRNP proteins alone contains the specificity required for recognition of the corresponding snRNAs.

Detection of HIV-Homologous DNA and RNA in Systemic Lupus Erythematosus

E. F. Krapf, W. Leitmann, M. Herrmann, and J. R. Kalden

Institute for Clinical Immunology, Dept. of Int. Med. III, University of Erlangen-Nürnberg, Erlangen, FRG

We recently reported the isolation of high molecular weight DNA from plasma of patients with systemic lupus erythematosus (SLE) [1]. Molecular cloning showed the presence of DNA with homology to the *gag-pol* region of HIV 1 (referred to as clone E 6). Transfection of plasma nucleic acids (PNA) into a human B cell line from a healthy donor (B 62) resulted in the induction of alterations commonly seen in cells infected by retroviruses. The cells transfected with PNA (B 62/SLE) showed morphological and physiological alterations absent in B 62. Besides syncitia formation, B 62/SLE cells express additional surface epitopes detected by immuno fluorescence using an antiserum against feline leucemia virus (FeLV) and by Western blot analysis with SLE patients' sera. Additional myristylated proteins were found in B 62/SLE as compared to B 62, with molecular weights similar to those in HIV-infected cells (Fig. 1).

Northern blots using E 6-DNA as probe provided evidence for retroviral mRNA production and suggested the presence of genomic viral RNA in B 62/SLE. Within the detection limits of Southern blotting, proviral sequences were found in *episomal* DNA of B 62/SLE cells but not in B 62. Southern blots from total genomic DNA gave possitive results in B 62 and B 62/SLE possibly resulting from a crossreactivity of E 6 with the endogenous human retrovirus PL 1 (Fig. 2).

In conclusion, these results suggest the presence of physiologically *active* retroviral nucleic acids in B 62/SLE and SLE patients plasma. Whether these nucleic acids are of exo- or endogenous origin needs further investigation.

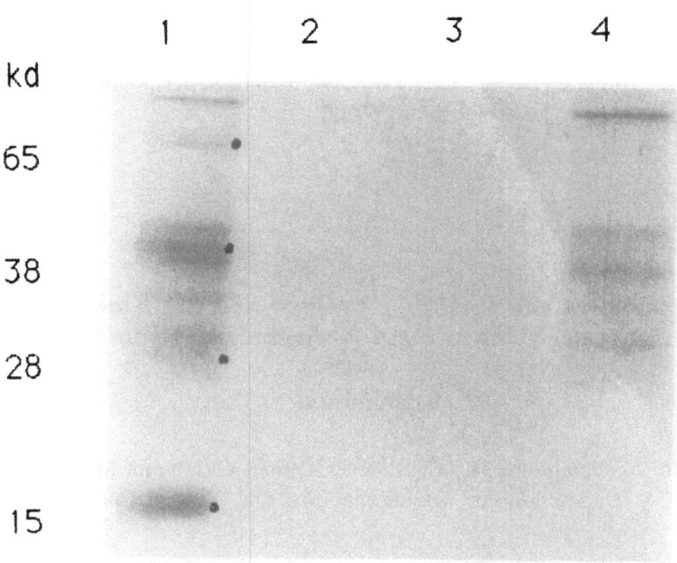

Fig. 1. The SDS-PAGE of ³H-myristate labelled proteins in B 62/SLE (lane 1), B 62 (lane 4) and in the PEG precipitated supernatants of B 62/SLE (lane 2: 5% PEG, lane 3: 20% PEG). Dots indicate proteins unique in B 62/SLE cells

```
E 6     1    GATCT GCCTT CCTGC AAGGG AAG  C CAGTG GACTT TTCT  CAGAG CAGCC AAGAG TCTGC
                       *               *     *    *        *     * *    * **
HIV 1        GATCT GCCTT CCTAC AAGGG AAGGC CAG  G GAATT TTCTT CAGAG CAGAC CAGAC CCAAC
                                                                                *
PL 1                                                                     AA TCTGC


E 6     60   CAT CACCA GAACA GCTGG TAGAA GACAA CAACT CCGTC TCAGA ACGCA GGA  C CGATA
                 **         *   **     *             **      *        *
HIV 1        AGCCC CACCA GAAGA G  GG TAGA  GACAA CAACT CCCCC TCAGA A GCA GGAGC CGATA
                *          **   ** *        *   *  *  *  ** *


PL 1         CAG CACCA GAACT TCTGA AA  AA GATAA AAAAT TTGTT TC


E 6     120  GA A      C TGTAT C TT  AACTT CCATC AGATC ATTCG GC AACGG AGC  157
                 * * *****       *  *         *          *
HIV 1        GACAA GGAAC TGTAT CCTTT AACTT CCCTC AGATC ACTC
```

Fig. 2. The homology of E 6 to the proviral genome of HIV 1 an to the endogenous retrovirus PL 1

Reference

1. KRAPF, F. E., HERRMANN, M., LEITMANN, W., KALDEN, J. R.: Clin. Exp. Immunol. (in press)

Heterogeneity of the Ro(SSA) Antigen and the Autoanti-Ro(SSA) Response: Evidence for 4 Antigenically Distinct Forms

M. Reichlin and Y. Itoh

University of Oklahoma Health Sciences Center, Oklahoma Medical Research Foundation, Oklahoma City, OK 73104, USA

Precipitating antibodies to the Ro(SSA) antigen occur in 40% of systemic lupus erythematosus (SLE) patients and 40–70% of patients with primary SJÖGREN's Syndrome. Previous work has shown that lymphocytes contain 2 Ro(SSA) antigens with protein moieties of 60 kD and 52 kD M.W. (J. Exp. Med. **167**, 1560–1571, 1988). We have reported that red cells contain 2 analogous but antigenically distinct Ro(SSA) molecules of M.W. 60 kD and 54 kD (J. Clin. Invest. **83**, 1293–1298, 1989). Of 43 sera with precipitating anti-Ro(SSA), some bind only one of the 4 isoforms in Western blot analysis. Moreover 42 of the 43 anti-Ro(SSA) bind 1 or more of the 4 Ro(SSA) isoforms. 29 sera react with RBC 60 kD Ro(SSA), 28 with Ly 60 kD Ro(SSA), 20 with RBC 54 kD Ro(SSA) and 16 with Ly 52 kD Ro(SSA). Since 15 of 16 sera reactive with Ly 52 kD Ro(SSA) also react with RBC 54 kD Ro(SSA), we postulate that these two molecules are structurally and antigenically related. Similarly 14 sera reacted only with the RBC and Ly 60 kD Ro(SSA) molecules suggesting an antigenic and structural relationship between them. Affinity isolation of antibodies to the various isoforms confirmed the antigenic relationship of the RBC and lymphocyte 60 kD forms of Ro(SSA) and similarly the antigenic relationship of the RBC 54 kD and lymphocyte 52 kD forms. Finally, this heterogeneity of Ro(SSA) is relevant to the anti-Ro(SSA) response as SLE sera with-Ro(SSA) and anti-nRNP all react better with RBC 60 kD Ro(SSA) than the RBC 54 kD Ro(SSA) in Western blot. Conversely, SLE sera with anti-Ro(SSA) and anti-La(SSB) precipitions react preferentially with RBC 54 kD Ro(SSA) over RBC 60 kD Ro(SSA) in Western blot in 90% of instances. These differences in antigenic fine specificity are being correlated with clinical phenomena.

Molecular Cloning of Ki Antigen C DNA and Enzyme-Linked-Immunosorbent-Assay for Anti-Ki Using Recombinant Ki

Y. Takasaki[1], M. Shibata[2], K. Shimada[3], T. Nikaidou[3], Y. Nishida[3], M. Sakamoto[1], H. Hashimoto[1], and S. Hirose[1]

[1] Juntendo University, Tokyo 113,
[2] Med. Bio. Lab.
[3] Aichi Cancer Center, Nagoya, Japan

In 1981, Tojo et al. firstly reported anti-Ki antibody and showed its clinical significance in lupus patients. But the characteristics of Ki antigen have not been well defined. In this report, we attempted to isolate the cDNA for Ki to elucidate the structure and function of this antigen, and establish enzyme-linked-immunosorbent-assay (ELISA) for anti-Ki antibodies using recombinant-antigen.

A cDNA clone (pb-Ki-1) for the Ki antigen was isolated from a cDNA library of bovine retina by using anti-Ki serum obtained from lupus patients. Using pb-Ki-1 as a probe, human full-length Ki cDNA clone (λ h-Ki-10) was also isolated from a $a$gt11 libraly of placenta mRNA. The sequence predicted a protein of 254 amino acids (M.W. 29508) with highly hydrophilic and weakly acidic characters. The purified bacterial product of pb-Ki (b-Na-X) was specifically reacted with anti-Ki sera in double immunodiffusion and immunoblotting and reactions were specifically inhibited by adsorption both with b-NA-X and Ki antigen purified from rabbit thymus extract.

Using b-NA-X as an antigen, ELISA for anti-Ki antibodies was established, Fifty µl (10 µl/ml) of antigen solution was added to a well of Immunoplate II (Nunc) to coat the antigen, and after sera (1 : 300) were reacted, reactions were detected by alkaline phosphatase labeled anti-human IgG. This system was specifically reacted with anti-Ki standard sera. When sera from patients with various rheumatic diseases were tested, anti-Ki antibodies were frequently detected in patients with lupus (14.4% out of 111) compared with patients with other dieseases (PSS 3.3%, PM/DM 6.6%, RA 6.0%, SjS 4.0%). In SLE, the frequencies of pericarditis and pleuritis were significantly high in patients with anti-Ki. Those results suggested that ELISA using recombinant Ki antigen was useful for the diagnosis of lupus reacting with anti-Ki antibodies specifically.

Antibodies to Nuclear Lamin C in Chronic Hepatitis Delta Virus Infection

J. Wesierska-Gadek[1], E. Penner[2], E. Hitchman[2], and G. Sauermann[1]

[1]Institute of Tumorbiology-Cancer Research and
[2]1st Department of Gastroenterology and Hepatology, University of Vienna, Vienna, Austria

The hepatitis delta virus is a defective RNA virus, dependent in its replication and infection on help provided by the hepatitis B virus. In this study we show that a majority of sera from patients with chronic hepatitis delta virus infection contain antibodies reacting exclusively with type C of the nuclear lamins. This antigen target was localized by immunofluorescence and identified in immunoblotting experiments, using different subnuclear fractions as antigen source.

The presence of antibodies solely recognizing nuclear lamin C is intriguing considering the primary structure of the nuclear lamins. Lamin C of 60 kD and lamin A of 70 kD molecular weight, occurring in equal amounts in the nuclear envelope, share extensive sequence homologies. Accordingly, antibodies observed in other autoimmune diseases, as in systemic rheumatic disorders or in chronic lupoid hepatitis (1), reacted with both, nuclear lamin A and lamin C. It appears that the presently described novel autoantibody associated with chronic hepatitis delta virus infection is recognizing an epitope in the carboxy-terminal region of nuclear lamin C.

References

1. WESIERSKA-GADEK, J., PENNER, E., HITCHMAN, E., SAUERMANN, G. (1988): Clin. Immunol. Immunopathol. **49**, 107–115

Sitzungsberichte der Heidelberger Akademie der Wissenschaften
Mathematisch-naturwissenschaftliche Klasse

Die Jahrgänge bis 1921 einschließlich erschienen im Verlag von Carl Winter, Universitätsbuchhandlung in Heidelberg, die Jahrgänge 1922–1933 im Verlag Walter de Gruyter & Co. in Berlin, die Jahrgänge 1934–1944 bei der Weißschen Universitätsbuchhandlung in Heidelberg. 1945, 1946 und 1947 sind keine Sitzungsberichte erschienen.

Ab Jahrgang 1948 erscheinen die „Sitzungsberichte" im Springer-Verlag.

Inhalt des Jahrgangs 1984:
1. R. Lüst. Extraterrestrische Astronomie. DM 17,–.
2. F. Leonhardt. Zu den Grundfragen der Ästhetik bei Bauwerken. DM 12,–.
3. Ch. Rüchardt. Die Bindung zwischen Kohlenstoffatomen, das Rückgrat der Organischen Chemie, und ihre Grenzen. DM 12,80.
4. J. Peiffer. Zur Neuropathologie der Nebenwirkungen nervenärztlicher Therapie. DM 18,–.
5. F. Linder. Geistige Grundlagen der chirurgischen Therapie. DM 14,–.

   Medizinische Anthropologie. Herausgegeben von E. Seidler. Supplement. Geb. DM 76,–.

   W.-W. Höpker. Mißbildungen. Interrelationen, Assoziationen und diagnostische Validität. Supplement. Geb. DM 74,–.

Inhalt des Jahrgangs 1985:
1. H. A. Staab. Zur Entstehung des Neuen in den Naturwissenschaften – dargestellt an einem Beispiel der Chemiegeschichte. DM 16,50.
2. S. Sambursky. Proklos, Präsident der platonischen Akademie, und sein Nachfolger, der Samaritaner Marinos. DM 13,–.
3. R. Haas. AIDS – Ein Virusinfekt des Immunsystems. DM 21,50.
4. F. Räbiger. Beiträge zur Strukturtheorie der Grothendieck-Räume. DM 39,50.
5. W. Kaiser. Entwicklungslinien der Breitbandkommunikation. DM 22,–.

   Pathogenese. Herausgegeben von H. Schipperges. Supplement. Geb. DM 88,–.

   E. Hinz. Human Helminthiases in the Philippines. Supplement. Geb. DM 98,–.

   T. Cremer. Von der Zellenlehre zur Chromosomentheorie. Supplement. Geb. DM 135,–.

Inhalt des Jahrgangs 1986:
1. W. Doerr. Hat das Menschengeschlecht eine biologische Zukunft? DM 22,50.
2. G. Schettler. Der Stoffwechsel der Plasmalipoproteine und seine Bedeutung für die Pathogenese der Arteriosklerose. DM 38,–.
3. A. Fröhlich. Tame Representations of Local Weil Groups and of Chain Groups of Local Principal Orders. DM 55,–.
4. W. Doerr. Pathologie in Heidelberg. Stufen nach 1945. DM 14,80.